IT ONLY LAUGHS WHEN I HURT

An

IN THE BLEACHERS

Collection of Painfully Funny Sports Injury Cartoons

(Vol. 1)

BWAAA-HA-HA-HA-HA-HA-HA-HAAA!!

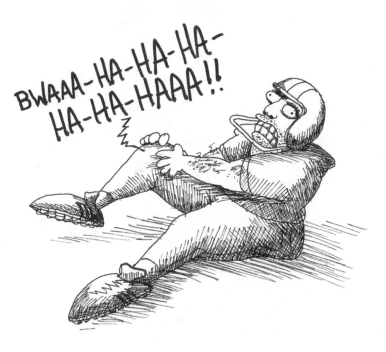

IT ONLY
LAUGHS
WHEN I
HURT

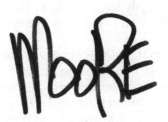

ACKLEY BOOKS

An infinitesimal imprint of an inconceivably ginormous secret publishing company

It Only Laughs When I Hurt:
An *In the Bleachers* Collection of Painfully Funny Sports Injury Cartoons
(Vol. 1)

 For information, address Ackley Books, 297 W Thornberry Drive, Boise, ID 83702.

ISBN 978-0-578-42004-2

Cover design by Blue Canary Books LLC
Cover art © 2019 by Steve Moore

>First Edition<

Dedicated to Athletic Trainers

The unsung heroes of sports medicine ...
who nevertheless seem to have an unhealthy obsession with rolls of
athletic tape.

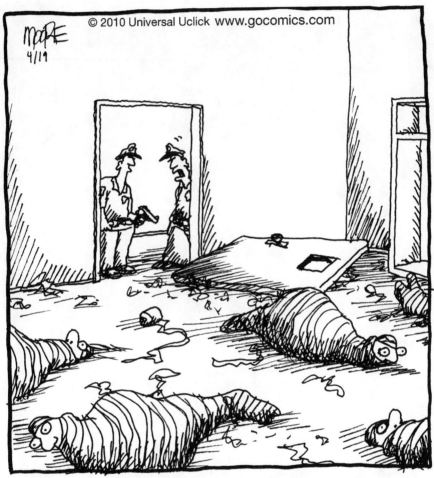

© 2010 Universal Uclick www.gocomics.com

"Same tragic story ... A disgruntled athletic trainer bursts into the locker room and starts taping players at random ... "

"Same tragic story ... A disgruntled athletic trainer bursts into the locker room and starts taping players at random."

PROLOGUE

I know what you're thinking: Why compile a collection of cartoons that lampoon sports injuries?

One reason is that sports medicine professionals - especially athletic trainers - asked me to do it. And I'm a fairly accommodating guy. The other reasons are more personal.

I was 7 when I first got hurt in sports. My dad was hitting grounders to me and a baseball smacked my shin, the most sensitive bone in the entire body. I cried, so Dad told a joke to distract me from the pain: "Why did the carpenter keep hitting himself in the head with a hammer? ... Because it felt good when he stopped." I laughed for a couple seconds, then I cried some more.

But Dad taught me a nifty formula: injury + sick humor = temporary pain relief. I used that formula often in my 30-plus years of *In the Bleachers*. (My archive has more than 1,000 injury cartoons, which is why this book is in two volumes.)

And then there are my knees. In college, I tore the weak and useless ACLs in both joints. It hurt worse than childbirth! (I'm pretty sure.) So I figured my painful knee experience gave me the right to joke about sports injuries. It's like if you're mauled by a psychopathic schnauzer you can joke about it. But if you've never been mauled by a psychopathic schnauzer you can't joke about it. Or something like that.

Anyway, I used my pain for gain and embarked with my dad's nifty formula on a mission of mercy. So if you got whacked by the wide world of hurt, I hope the cartoons in this book provide at least a couple seconds of pain relief.

- STEVE MOORE

© 2000 Universal Press Syndicate
MOORE
6-20

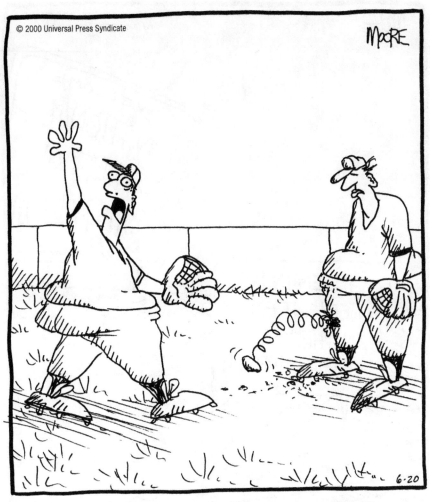

"Time! Steve's knee popped out again!"

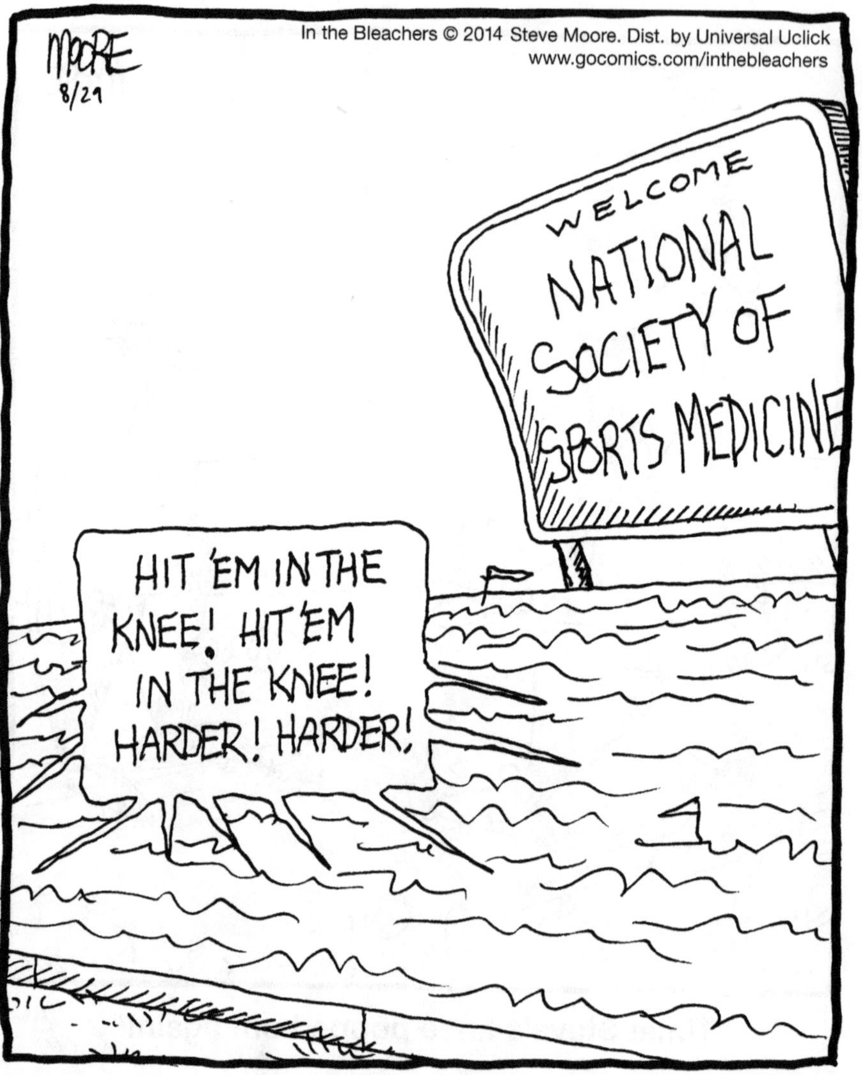
MOORE 8/29
In the Bleachers © 2014 Steve Moore. Dist. by Universal Uclick
www.gocomics.com/inthebleachers
WELCOME
NATIONAL SOCIETY OF SPORTS MEDICINE
HIT 'EM IN THE KNEE! HIT 'EM IN THE KNEE! HARDER! HARDER!

© 2000 Universal Press Syndicate
MOORE
10-18
www.uexpress.com

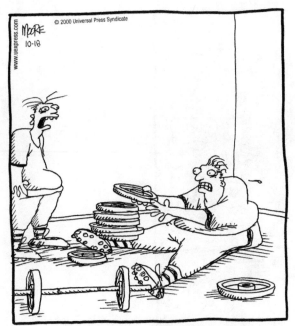

"I don't know if that's such a good idea, Louie. Doc said to keep weight off the ankle until it heals."

8-1
© 2001 Universal Press Syndicate
MOORE
www.ucomics.com
CAREERS IN SPORTS BROAD-CASTING

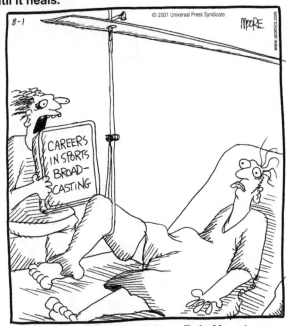

"Sorry about the knee injury, Bob. Your teammates chipped in and bought you a book to read while you're recovering."

MOORE
6-1
© 2000 Universal Press Syndicate www.uexpress.com
POP!!
OUCH!

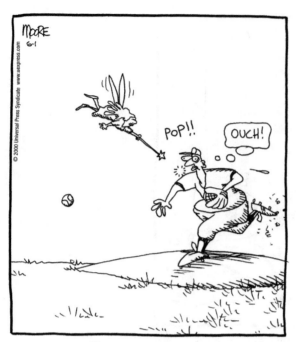

The rotator cuff fairy.

9-4
MOORE
www.ucomics.com
© 2002 Universal Press Syndicate

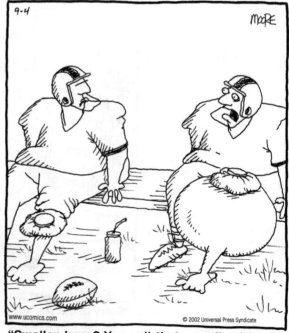

"Swollen knee? You call *that* a swollen knee?"

MOORE
2/6
In the Bleachers © 2014 Steve Moore. Dist. by Universal Uclick
www.gocomics.com/inthebleachers

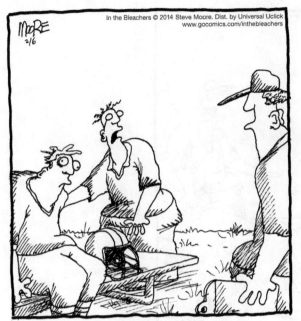

"I don't believe it's a concussion, but out of an abundance of caution, I've called for an attorney."

12-16
MOORE
www.uexpress.com
© 1998 Universal Press Syndicate

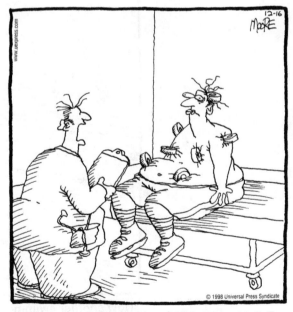

"Lungs, normal. Heart, normal. Kidneys, normal. For the life of me, I can't figure out where your pain is coming ... wait. Do you play hockey?"

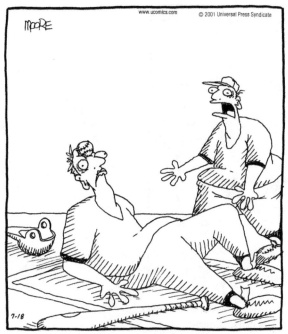

www.ucomics.com
© 2001 Universal Press Syndicate
MOORE
7-18

"Where does it hurt?"

www.ucomics.com
© 2002 Universal Press Syndicate
MOORE
2-7

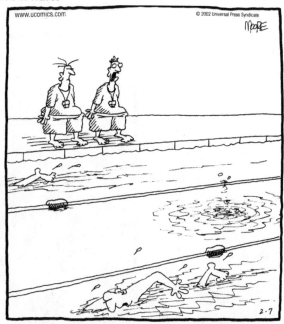

"Now *another* swimmer's been dragged under, screaming, right in the middle of a race. I'm telling you, Floyd, something's down there."

IN THE BLEACHERS

BY STEVE MOORE

MARATHON!! VEND-O-MAT
FRESH!! KNEE CARTILAGE
SHIN SPLINT REPELLENT
AUXILIARY LUNG
CRAMP -B- GONE!
MOORE
8-17
www.gocomics.com

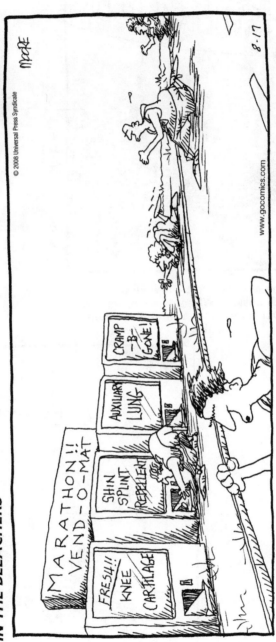

© 2007 Universal Press Syndicate
ANNUAL
ATHLETIC TRAINER
ANKLE-TAPING CHAMPIONSHIP
MOORE
www.gocomics.com
8-1

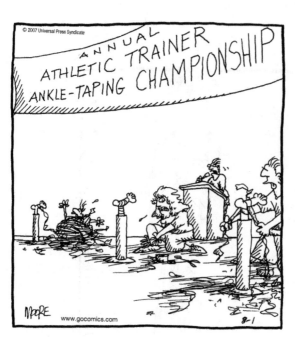

"Seven seconds flat – a new world record! ... Wait. Whoa! How ironic is that? Our champion sprained her own ankle."

© 2007 Universal Press Syndicate
IT'S HIS K-N-E-E AND HE'S TORN HIS L-I-G-A-M-E-N-T-S.
HELLOOOO. I CAN SPELL!
www.gocomics.com
MOORE
7-14

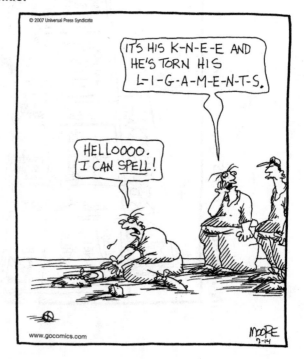

MOORE
CLAP!
CLAP!
CLAP!
© 2005 Universal Press Syndicate
2/1

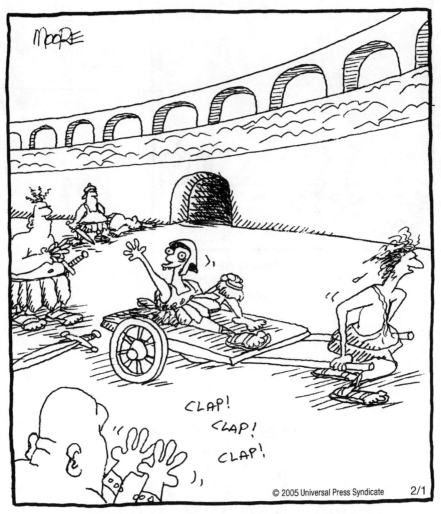

After the brief display of sportsmanship, the gladiators resumed fighting to the death, while Anthony embarked on the long road to rehabilitation from torn knee ligaments.

In the Bleachers © 2012 Steve Moore. Dist. by Universal Uclick
MOORE
1/23
www.gocomics.com/inthebleachers

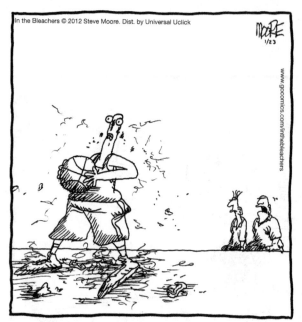

"Usually, with older players, the legs are the first to go. But in rare cases it's the hair, ears and nose."

© 1996 Universal Press Syndicate
MOORE
12-14
www.uexpress.com

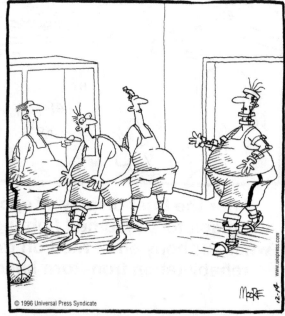

The other players were impressed with Vince's new state-of-the-art knee brace ... until Andy walked in.

JdsMOORE@AOL.COM
www.uexpress.com
© 1997 Universal Press Syndicate
MOORE
REX — DEAD
ANDY — DEAD
JULIUS — DEAD
XAVIOR — DEAD
TREVOR — DEAD
BOB — DEAD
DARIUS — BACK SPASMS
VIRGIL — DEAD
MARCUS — DEAD
SIDNEY — DEAD
11-29

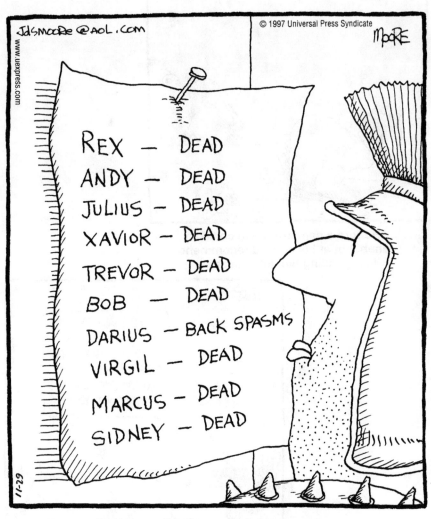

Roman gladiator injury reports.

In the Bleachers © 2015 Steve Moore. Dist. by Universal Uclick
www.gocomics.com/inthebleachers
MOORE
4/25

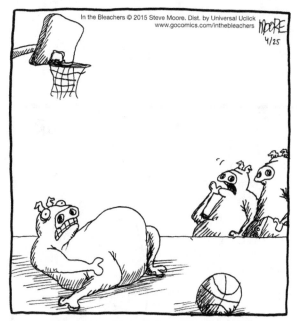

"He tore a hamstring. We could try rehab, but at his age, I'd recommend just grinding him into sausage."

MOORE
© 2007 Universal Press Syndicate
8-3
A MESSAGE FROM THE VIKINGS, SIRE. IT SAYS, 'WE'VE GOT SPIRIT! YES, WE DO! WE'VE GOT SPIRIT! HOW ABOUT YOU!?'
www.gocomics.com

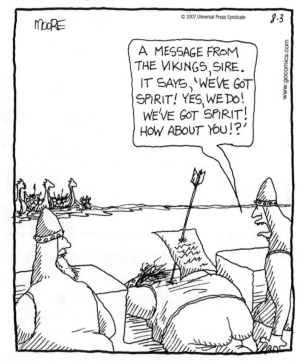

www.uexpress.com
© 2000 Universal Press Syndicate
MOORE
1-29
DANGER
WATCH OUT FOR WARNING SIGNS PLACED RIGHT IN THE MIDDLE OF THE SKI SLOPE.

© 1997 Universal Press Syndicate
www.uexpress.com
KEEP YOUR HEAD DOWN.
DON'T LISTEN TO HIM!!
JdsmooRe@AoL.com
MOORE
6-21

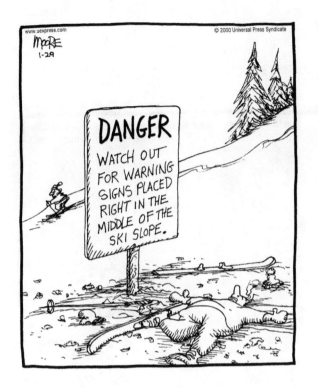

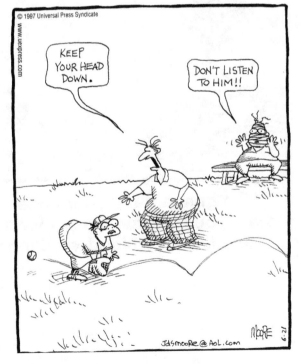

In the Bleachers © 2013 Steve Moore. Dist. by Universal Uclick
www.gocomics.com/inthebleachers
MOORE
7/13

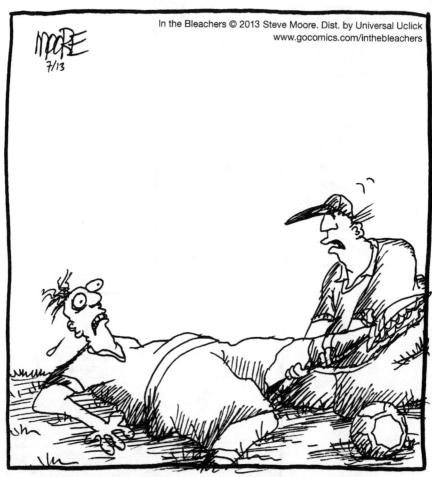

"I'm gonna bend your knee. If it hurts, I want you to scrunch up your face in agony and let out a blood-curdling scream."

MOORE
Jdsmoore @AoL.com
2-3
© 1998 Universal Press Syndicate www.uexpress.com

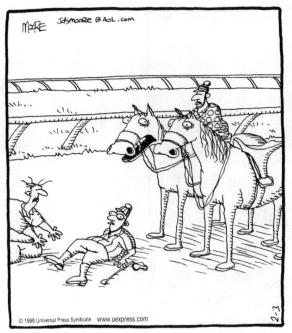

"It's his knee. If they have an ounce of compassion, they'll just shoot him."

DR. R. FLEM
THERAPIST
MARRIAGES,
FAMILIES,
DOUBLE-PLAY
COMBOS
MOORE
3-5
© 1999 Universal Press Syndicate
www.uexpress.com

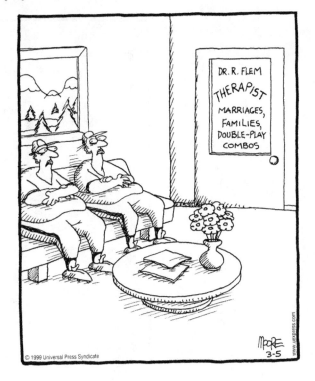

MOORE JdSMOORE@AOL.COM © 1998 Universal Press Syndicate www.uexpress.com
3-6

"I'm sorry. We tried everything. Your knee is dead."

3-29
© 2001 Universal Press Syndicate
PLAYER STATUS REPORTS
INJURED LIST
SUSPENDED LIST
INDICTED LIST
CONVICTED LIST
INCARCERATED LIST
MOORE
www.ucomics.com

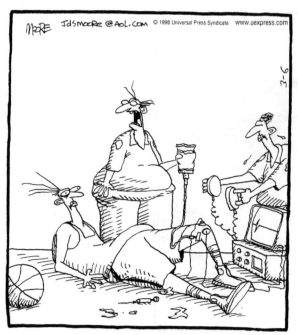

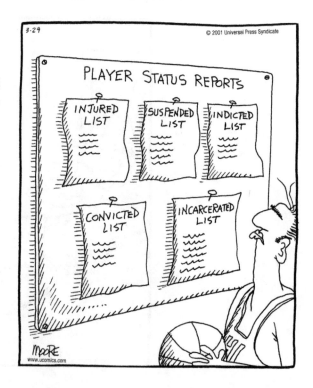

www.ucomics.com
WE NEED TO PUT YOU ON THE INJURED LIST TO MAKE ROOM ON THE ROSTER.
BUT I'M NOT HURT.
MOORE
© 2001 Universal Press Syndicate
10-30

www.ucomics.com
© 2001 Universal Press Syndicate
MOORE
11-22

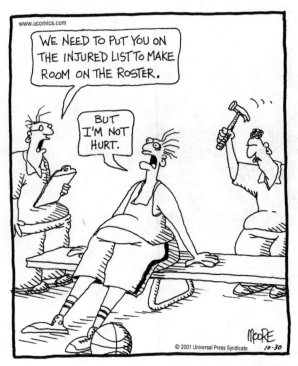

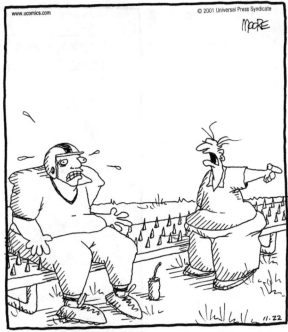

"Stop whining! If the guys on the field can play with pain, then you can sit with pain!"

SHIELD YOUR UDDER.
© 1999 Universal Press Syndicate
MOORE 9-22
www.uexpress.com

© 2003 Universal Press Syndicate
WHOA! LOOKS LIKE YOU THREW OUT YOUR ELBOW.
HERE IT IS!
MOORE
www.ucomics.com
5-12

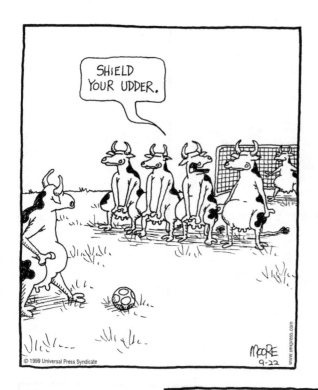

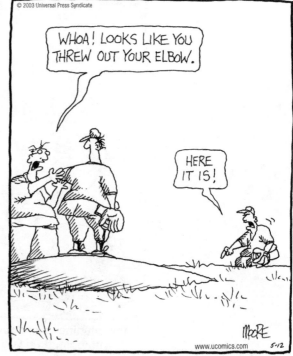

IN THE BLEACHERS

BY STEVE MOORE

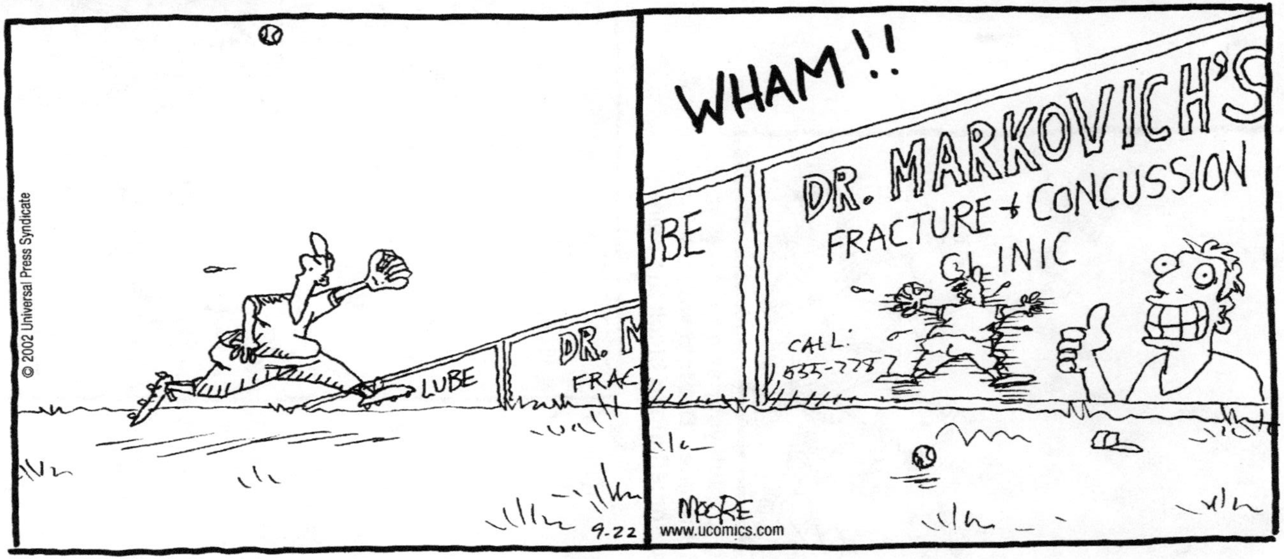

WHAM!!

DR. MARKOVICH'S
FRACTURE + CONCUSSION
CLINIC

CALL: 555-7787

LUBE

© 2002 Universal Press Syndicate

www.ucomics.com

MOORE
1/25 In the Bleachers © 2016 Steve Moore. Dist. by Universal Uclick
www.gocomics.com/inthebleachers

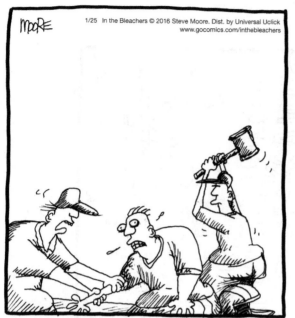

"I'm going to yank your arm to re-set your dislocated shoulder. But first we're going to give you something to block the pain."

© 2008 Universal Press Syndicate
www.gocomics.com
MOORE
HOW BAD IS IT?
HE'S GOT ISSUES WITH HIS MOTHER... I CAN'T PROMISE ANYTHING, BUT HE SHOULD BE BACK IN THE GAME BY THE SECOND HALF.
4-2

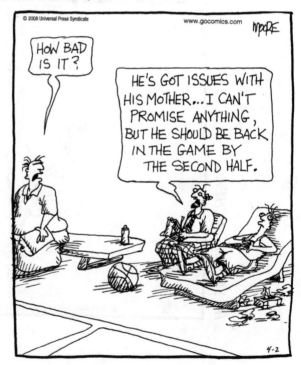

© 1998 Universal Press Syndicate
MOORE
6-18
www.uexpress.com

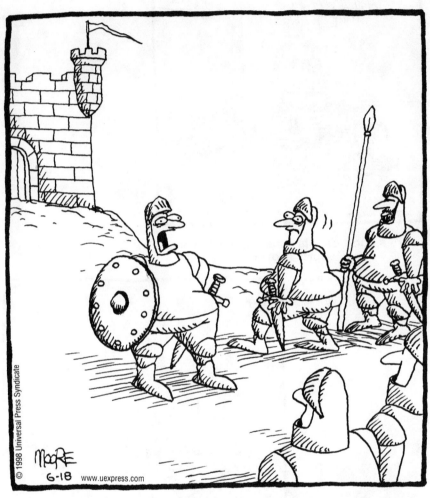

"Well, you just march right back to the castle and put one on. ... Anyone else not wearing a cup?"

© 2007 Universal Press Syndicate
WAAAAAAH!!
DAYCAR
11-12 www.gocomics.com
MOORE

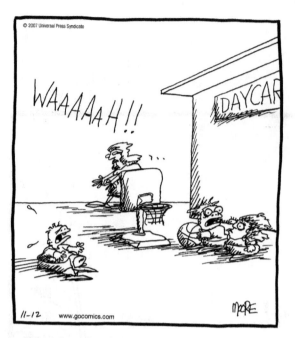

"It's a boo-boo! His career in professional sports is over!"

© 2010 Universal Uclick www.gocomics.com
MOORE
4/6

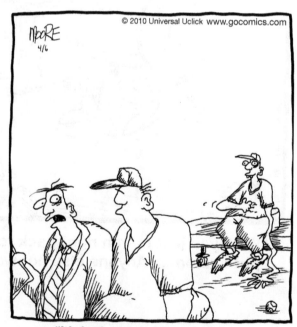

"It's bad, coach. Not only is your pitcher a belly itcher, but X-rays confirm that he's also got a rubber arm."

YOU'VE ABSORBED MANY PUNCHES IN YOUR BOXING CAREER. HAVE YOU SUFFERED PERMANENT DAMAGE?
COULD YOU REPEAT THE QUESTION?
YOU'VE ABSORBED MANY PUNCHES IN YOUR BOXING CAREER. HAVE YOU SUFFERED PERMANENT DAMAGE?
COULD YOU REPEAT THE QUESTION?
I'M GOING TO ASSUME YOUR ANSWER IS 'YES.' IS THAT OK?
COULD YOU REPEAT THE QUESTION?
3-1
MOORE

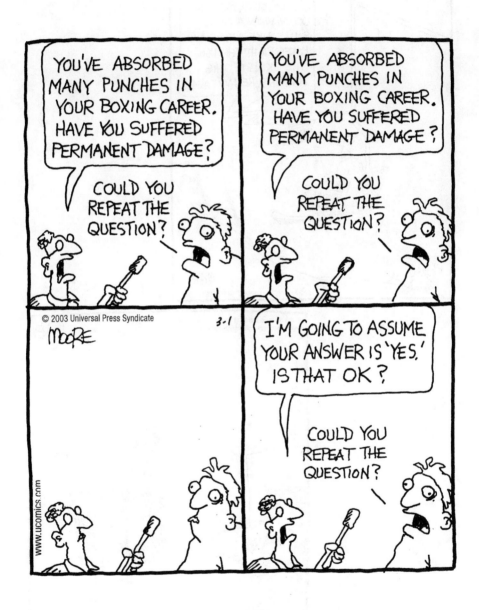

www.ucomics.com
...COMPOUND FRACTURES OCCUR WHEN A BONE SNAPS LIKE A TWIG AND POKES RIGHT THROUGH THE SKIN. IF THIS HAPPENS, REMAIN CALM...
MOORE
2-21
© 2003 Universal Press Syndicate

In the Bleachers © 2014 Steve Moore. Dist. by Universal Uclick
www.gocomics.com/inthebleachers
MOORE
6/16

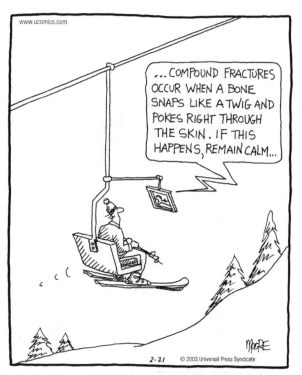

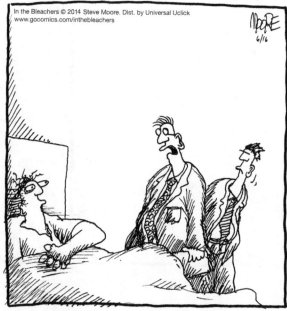

"The Tommy John surgery was a success! However, we need to go back in. Dr. Moore can't find his wedding ring."

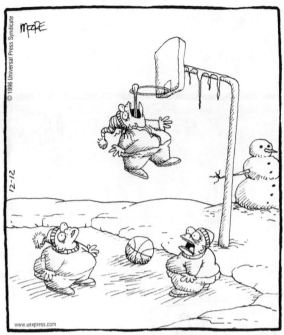

© 1996 Universal Press Syndicate
MOORE
12-12
www.uexpress.com

"Go get help."

In the Bleachers © 2002 Steve Moore. Dist. by Universal Uclick 1/10
MOORE

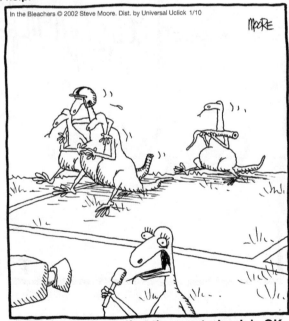

"Initial reports are that the quarterback is OK and will return in the second half. His tail, however, probably won't grow back in time for the playoffs."

In the Bleachers © 2015 Steve Moore. Dist. by Universal Uclick
www.gocomics.com/inthebleachers
MOORE 7/14
LEAVING
YOUR ATHLETIC PRIME
THANK YOU FOR VISITING!!

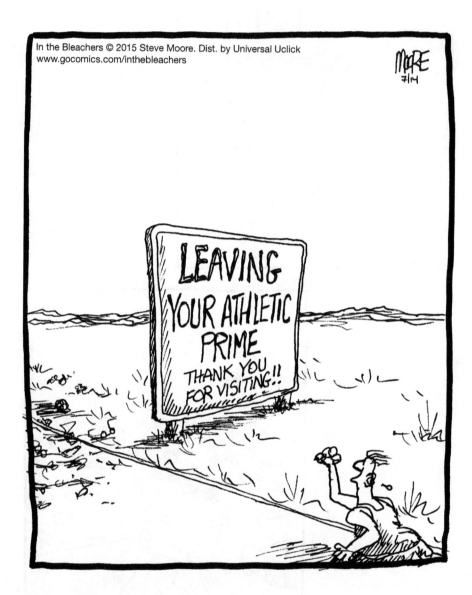

WHUMP!!
www.uexpress.com
© 1998 Universal Press Syndicate
MOORE 5-11

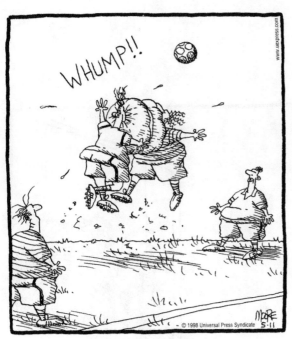

Two players collide, airbags inflate, and another soccer tragedy is averted.

www.uexpress.com
© 2000 Universal Press Syndicate
MOORE 8-23

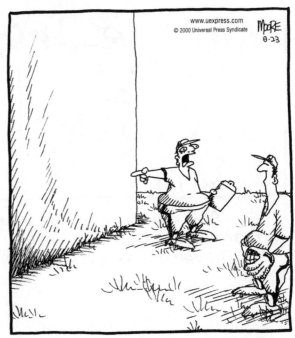

"Thayer! We need to open up a spot on the roster. Sprint head-first into that concrete wall."

www.gocomics.com
MOORE
11-27
ANNUAL
SPORTS
INJURY
AWARDS
© 2009 Universal Uclick

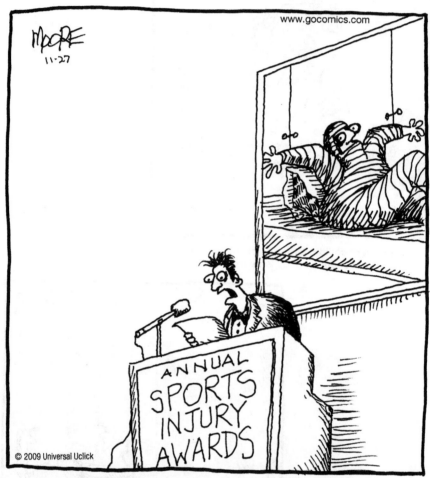

"... And the Outstanding Injury of the Year Award goes to — Dewey Taylor! ... Dewey joins us via video link ..."

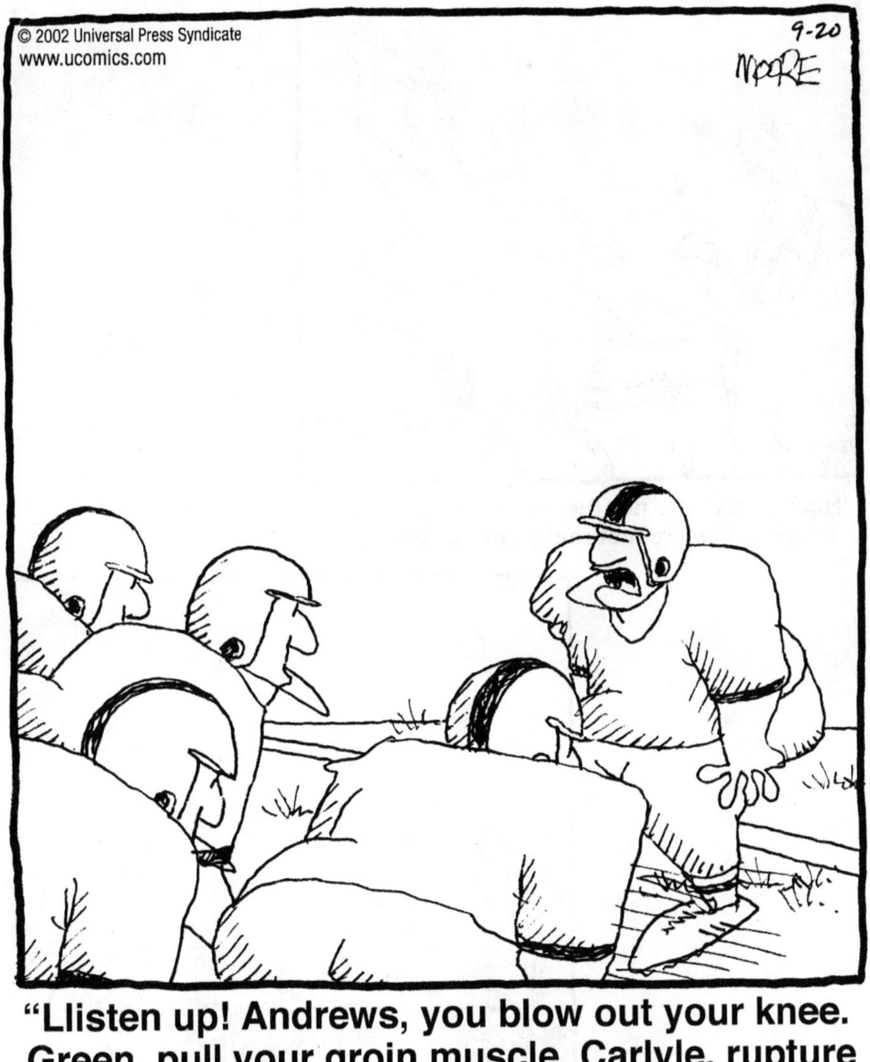

© 2002 Universal Press Syndicate
www.ucomics.com
9-20
MOORE

"Llisten up! Andrews, you blow out your knee. Green, pull your groin muscle. Carlyle, rupture your spleen. I'll drop back and get a concussion. ... Everyone else block."

© 2009 Universal Uclick
www.gocomics.com
MOORE
12-9

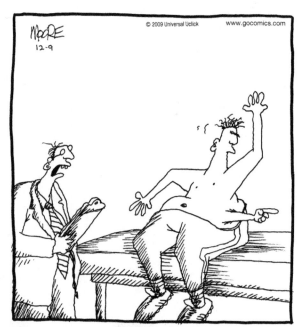

"Hip pointers are not the most serious sports injuries. They're just really embarrassing."

www.ucomics.com
© 2002 Universal Press Syndicate
MOORE
4-19

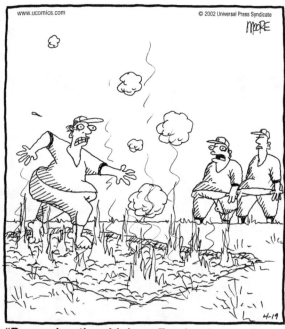

"Remember the old days, Frank, when a player would screw up and we'd say, 'Drop down and give me 20 push-ups'? ... This is more fun."

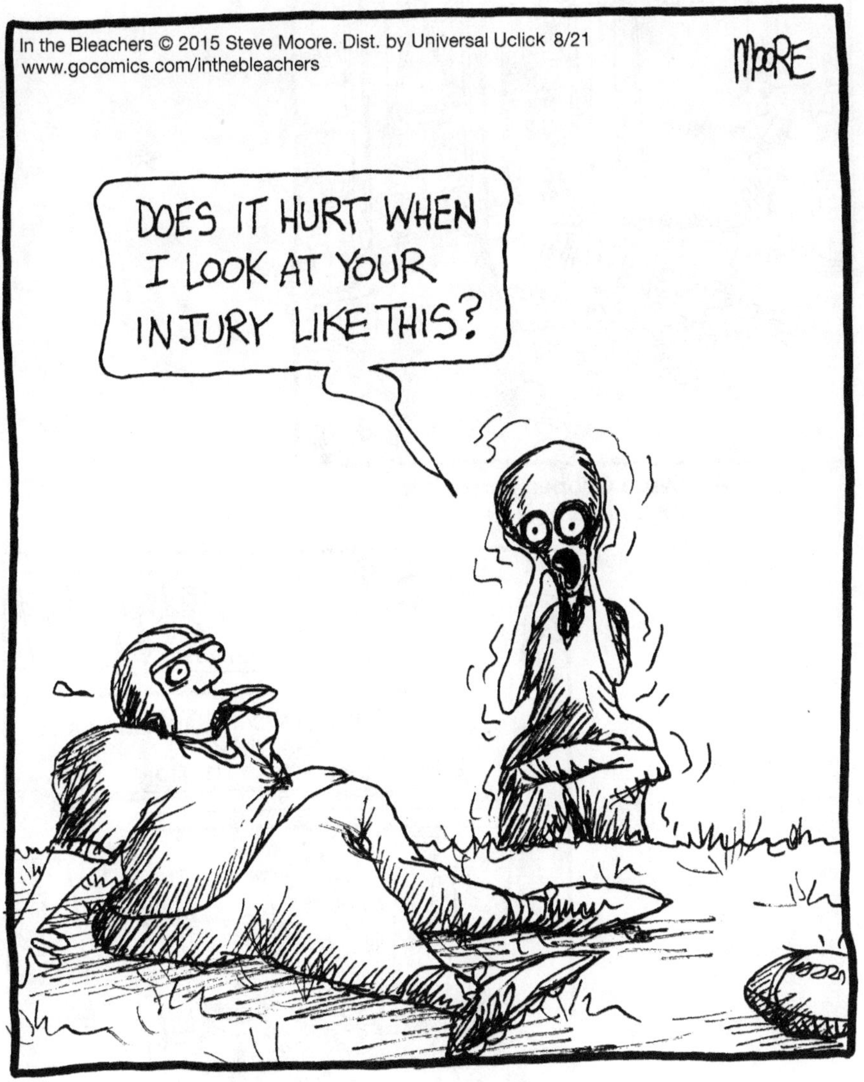
In the Bleachers © 2015 Steve Moore. Dist. by Universal Uclick 8/21
www.gocomics.com/inthebleachers
MOORE
DOES IT HURT WHEN I LOOK AT YOUR INJURY LIKE THIS?

www.ucomics.com
© 2001 Universal Press Syndicate
INJURED RESERVE
MOORE 1-22

"Reactivate Cooper. I need him for tonight's game."

VICTIMS OF SPORTS ILLUSTRATED
COVER JINX
HOSPITAL AND REHABILITATION
www.uexpress.com
MOORE 4-6
© 2000 Universal Press Syndicate

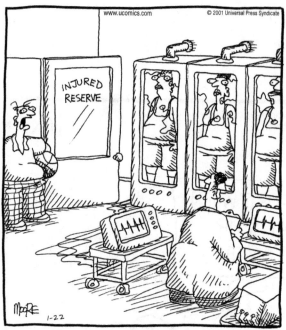

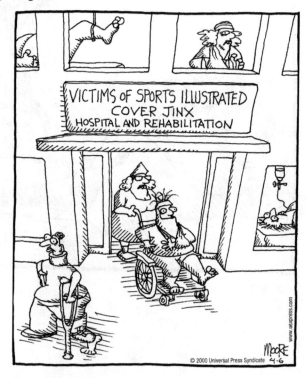

© 2000 Universal Press Syndicate
www.uexpress.com
7-24
MOORE
KNOCKED UNCONSCIOUS. BACK IN A JIFF!

© 2001 Universal Press Syndicate
www.ucomics.com
MOORE
ATHLETIC TRAINER
4-24

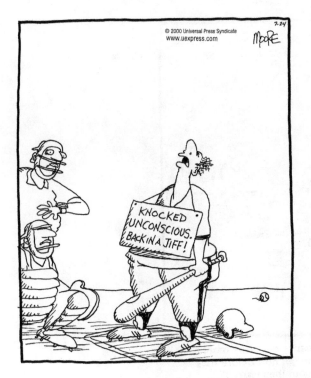

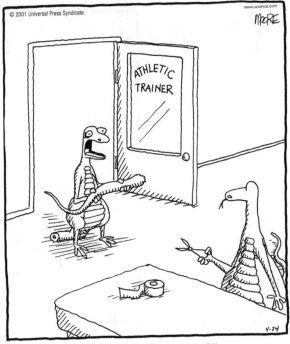

"Can you tape me up?"

MOORE
7-24
© 1997 Universal Press Syndicate www.uexpress.com

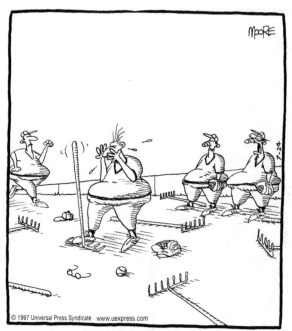

"It's negligence, man! How many more of us players have to get hurt before they do something about these rakes?"

MOORE
11-12
© 2002 Universal Press Syndicate

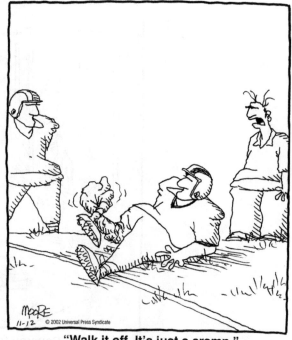

"Walk it off. It's just a cramp."

3-6
MOORE
www.uexpress.com
© 1999 Universal Press Syndicate
YEE-AAAH!
AAAAAH!
AAA-EEE!

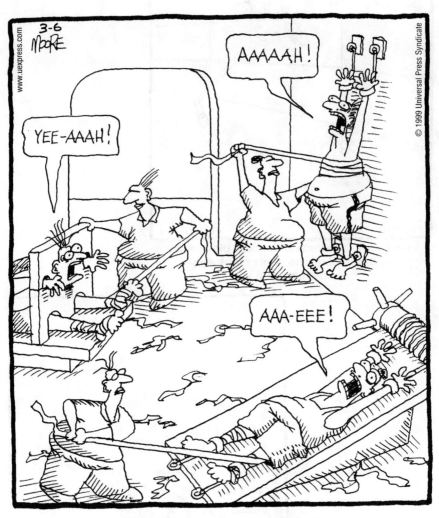

Athletic tape removal chamber.

MOORE
1-15
© 2002 Universal Press Syndicate
www.ucomics.com

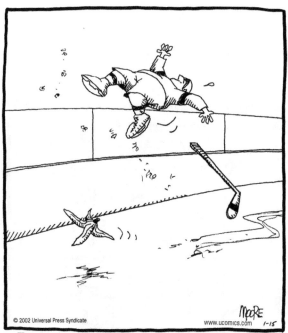

Every year, hundreds of hockey players are injured by banana peels carelessly tossed onto the ice.

MOORE
8-28
www.uexpress.com
© 2000 Universal Press Syndicate

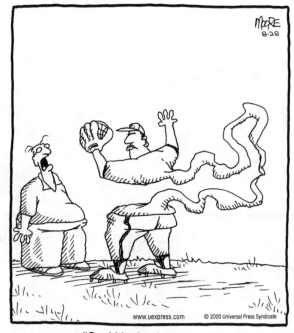

"Could be back spasms."

MOORE
8-11 © 2000 Universal Press Syndicate
www.uexpress.com

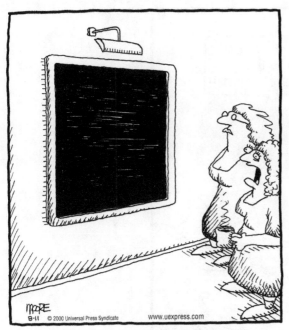

"My husband was a quarterback, but he retired because he kept getting concussions. Now he paints. This one's called 'Memories' ..."

© 2002 Universal Press Syndicate
NO, PHYLLIS, THAT'S INCORRECT. CAN ANYONE ELSE DEMONSTRATE THE PROPER WAY TO TAPE AN ANKLE?
www.ucomics.com
MOORE 1-24

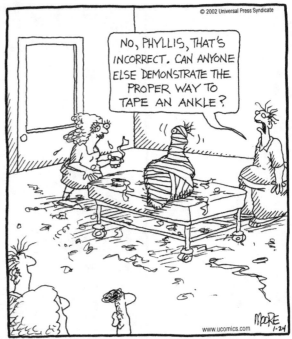

Freshman athletic trainers.

www.ucomics.com
MOORE
1-23
EXCUSE ME! I KNOW HOW TO DO THE HEIMLICH MANEUVER!!
© 2002 Universal Press Syndicate

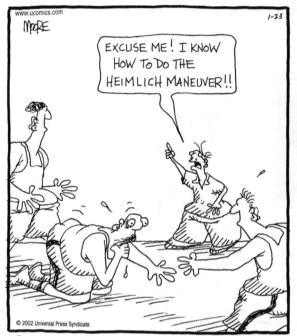

Cory is saved, and the game ball is recovered in relatively good condition.

MOORE
11-30

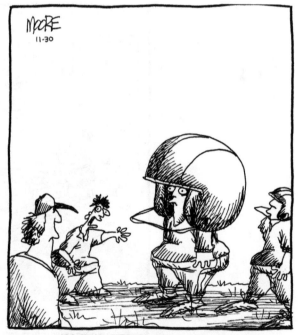

"Voila! ... Concussion-proof!"

9-24
www.gocomics.com
MOORE
AAAAAAAAH!!
© 2008 Universal Press Syndicate

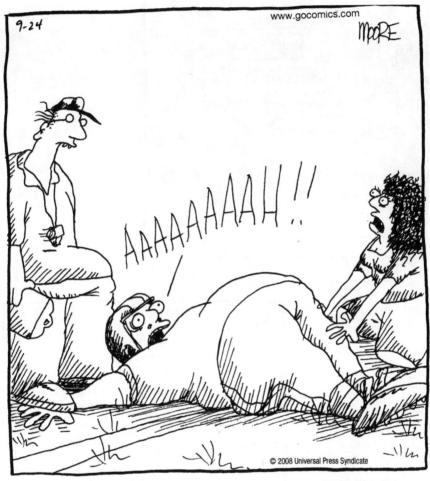

"The pain in his side indicates cracked ribs. The tender knee is possible ligament damage. And the screaming means you're standing on his hand."

www.ucomics.com
QUIT SQUIRMING!
ARE YOU CHEWING GUM? SPIT IT OUT!
DON'T SLOUCH!
WHERE'S MY PAIN MEDICINE?
MOORE
© 2004 Universal Press Syndicate
1-24

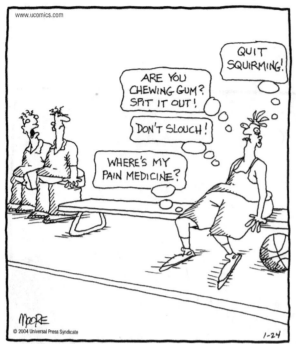

"I'm keeping Tony out of the game. He's still dealing with a few nagging injuries."

MOORE
3/21
In the Bleachers © 2014 Steve Moore. Dist. by Universal Uclick
www.gocomics.com/inthebleachers
90 MPH FASTBALL RIGHT IN THE KIDNEY #5

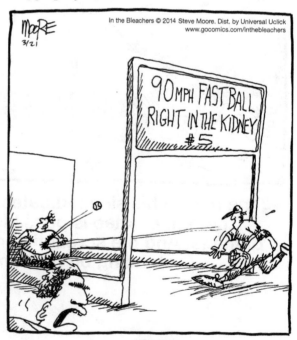

"Next!"

In the Bleachers © 2014 Steve Moore. Dist. by Universal Uclick
www.gocomics.com/inthebleachers
MOORE 4/3
YOU ARE HERE
HOSPITAL

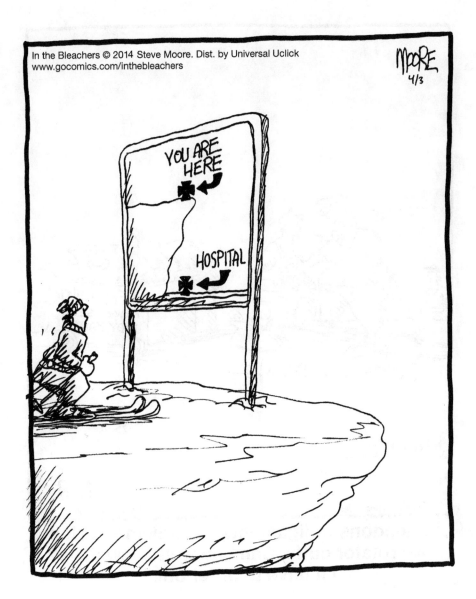

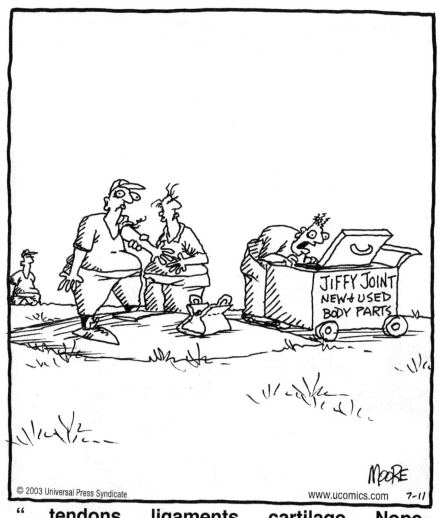

www.ucomics.com 7-11

"... tendons ... ligaments ... cartilage ... Nope.
No rotator cuffs. Can you wait a few days?
I'll have to order one."

© 2003 Universal Press Syndicate
9-19
MOORE
www.ucomics.com

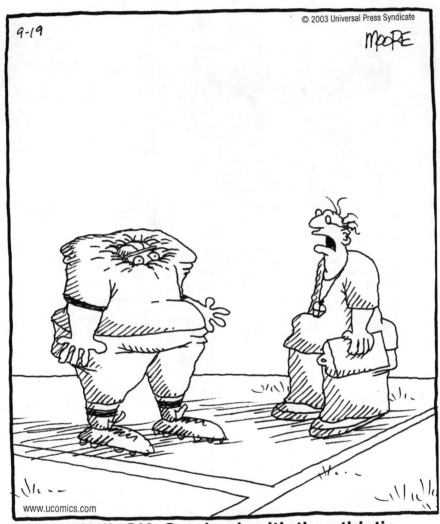

"Well, OK. Go check with the athletic trainer. ... But you'd better not be faking it just to avoid practice."

© 2002 Universal Press Syndicate
MOORE
11-29
www.ucomics.com

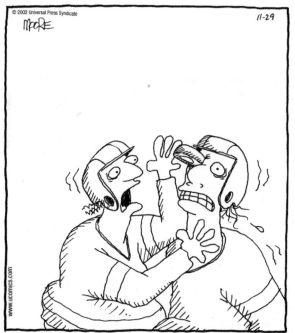

"Look up ... nothing ... nothing. ... Wait! Yes. You've got a hockey puck stuck in your eye."

6-25
© 2008 Universal Press Syndicate
MOORE
www.gocomics.com

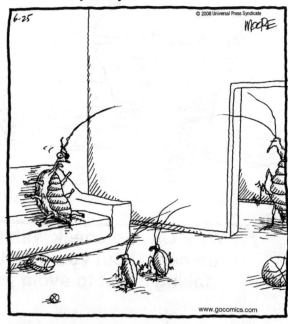

"When I played sports, dadgummit, we *never* came out of the game. If you got hurt, you'd just play with pain."

WHAT IS AN ISOSCELES TRIANGLE? IN WHAT YEAR DID TEDDY ROOSEVELT RIDE UP SAN JUAN HILL? WHO INVENTED DENTAL FLOSS? ...
IT'S PROBABLY A CONCUSSION. HE'S BEEN UNABLE TO ANSWER EVEN ONE QUESTION CORRECTLY.
MOORE 7-12
www.uexpress.com

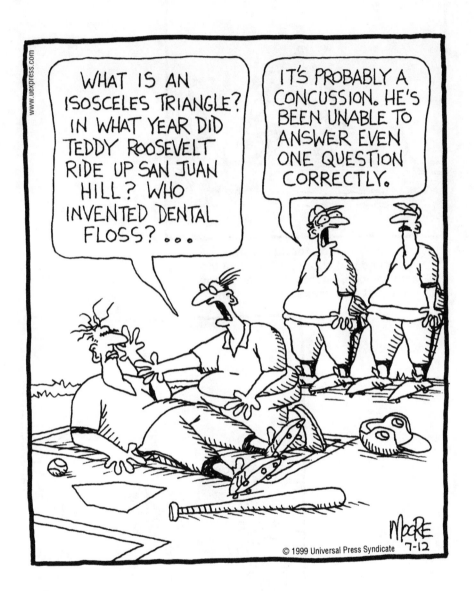

MOORE
5/28
In the Bleachers © 2014 Steve Moore. Dist. by Universal Uclick
www.gocomics.com/inthebleachers

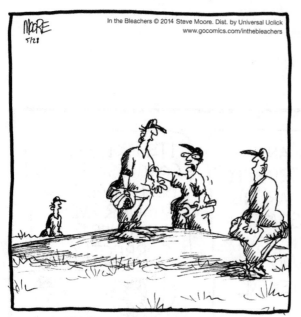

"Well, his rotator cuff is shot. I warned you about pitching him too many innings, but hey. What do I know? I'm just a transmission mechanic!"

MOORE
6/30
In the Bleachers © 2014 Steve Moore. Dist. by Universal Uclick
www.gocomics.com/inthebleachers
JOCK RASH -B- GONE

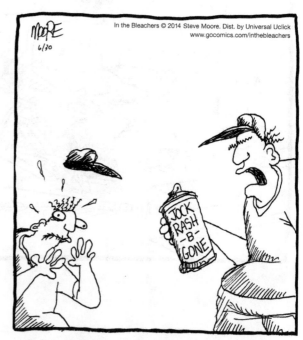

"My mistake. It says 'External Use Only' ..."

In the Bleachers © 2014 Steve Moore. Dist. by Universal Uclick
www.gocomics.com/inthebleachers
MOORE
7/10
PITBULLS

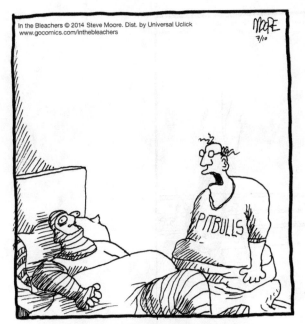

"Your teammates send best wishes. And management has decided to hire someone in a mascot outfit instead of having a live animal."

In the Bleachers © 2014 Steve Moore. Dist. by Universal Uclick
www.gocomics.com/inthebleachers
MOORE
10/11

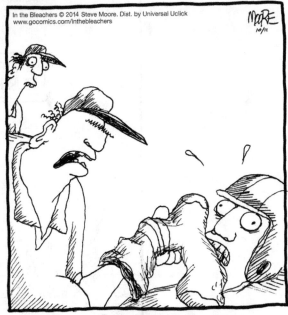

"I said 'smelling salts.' You brought me smelly socks! ... Well, it's working."

MOORE
3/28
In the Bleachers © 2015 Steve Moore. Dist. by Universal Uclick
www.gocomics.com/inthebleachers

"... Eight ... nine ... ten ...
Fight's over! He's squashed!!"

MOORE
1/31
In the Bleachers © 2015 Steve Moore. Dist. by Universal Uclick
www.gocomics.com/inthebleachers
YOU BLEW OUT YOUR KNEE.

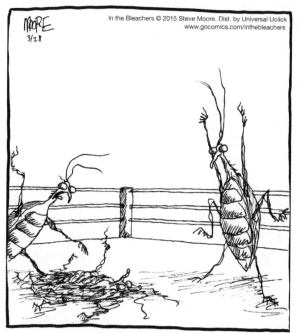

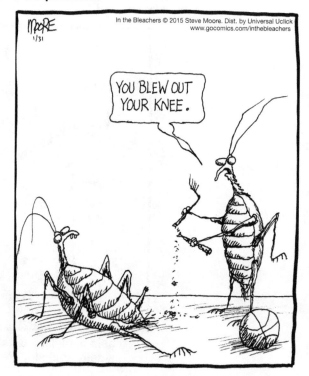

www.ucomics.com
© 2001 Universal Press Syndicate
MOORE
10-10

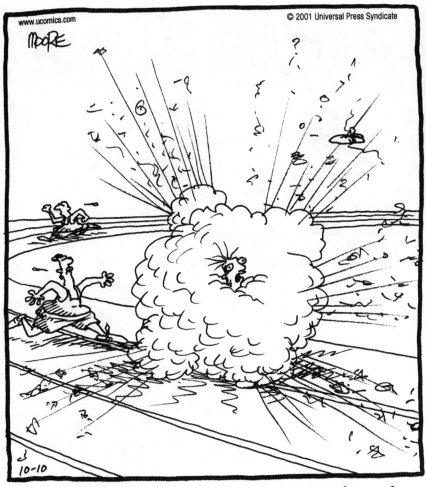

Ernie forgets to stretch out properly and simultaneously blows out his knees, ankles, shoulders, elbows, wrists, hips, and the joints on all 10 fingers.

In the Bleachers © 2014 Steve Moore. Dist. by Universal Uclick
www.gocomics.com/inthebleachers
MOORE 11/7
POOF!!

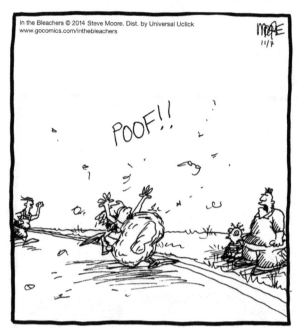

"This is the point in the marathon where runners 'hit the wall.' Fortunately, they have all been equipped with safety airbags."

In the Bleachers © 2015 Steve Moore. Dist. by Universal Uclick
www.gocomics.com/inthebleachers
MOORE 7/1
REALLY? NO ONE BROUGHT ANESTHETIC? THIS IS A TOMMY JOHN SURGERY! WELL, I GUESS HE'LL NEED TO JUST TOUGH IT OUT.

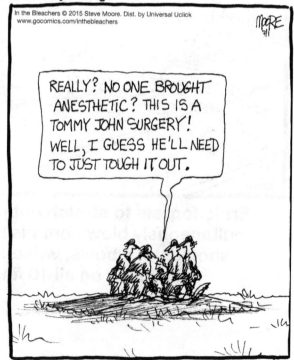

www.gocomics.com/inthebleachers
THUMP!
MOORE
6/23
In the Bleachers © 2015 Steve Moore. Dist. by Universal Uclick
FORE!!

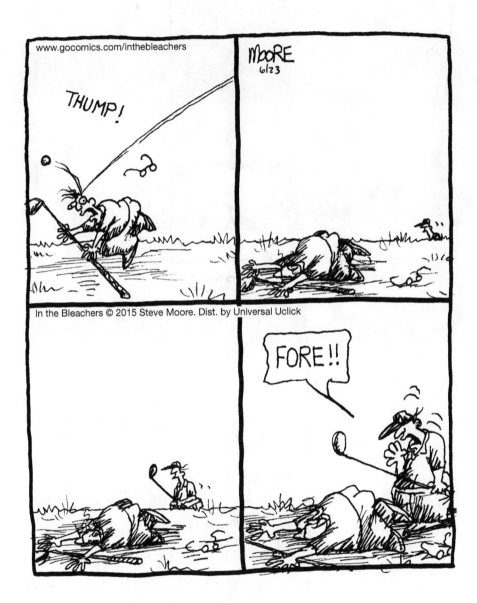

In the Bleachers © 2010 Steve Moore. Dist. by Universal Uclick
www.gocomics.com/inthebleachers
MOORE
1/17

“Get up. It’s just a crack. No yolk, no foul.”

In the Bleachers © 2015 Steve Moore. Dist. by Universal Uclick
www.gocomics.com/inthebleachers
MOORE
5/14
TOUCHED SOCCER BALL WITH MY HAND
DODGED WHEN I SHOULDA WEAVED
RIP
TOOK MY EYE OFF OF THE BALL
FORGOT TO DUCK

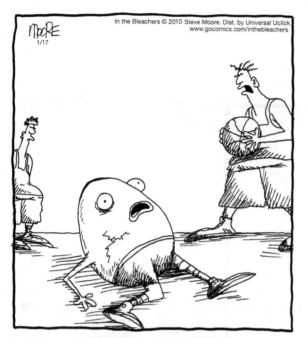

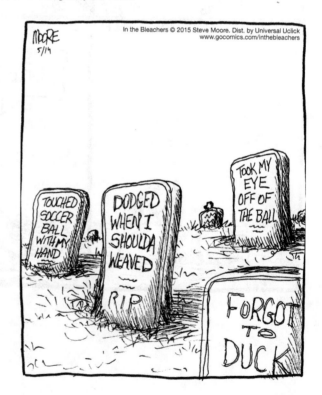

In the Bleachers © 2015 Steve Moore. Dist. by Universal Uclick
www.gocomics.com/inthebleachers
MOORE 4/10
BEGONE!!
DEWEY, YOU FOOL! THAT'S A SHIN SPLINTS HEALER! YOU NEED A LEG CRAMP HEALER!!

In the Bleachers © 2015 Steve Moore. Dist. by Universal Uclick
www.gocomics.com/inthebleachers
MOORE 5/19

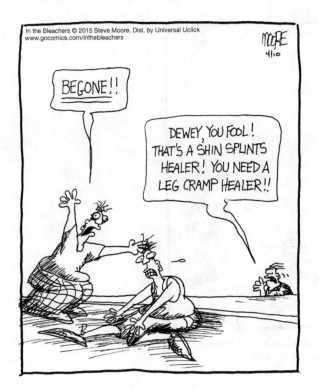

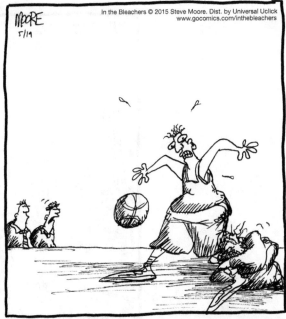

"Hey, I'm an athletic trainer. I can deal with leg cramps, but I know nothing about leg gramps!"

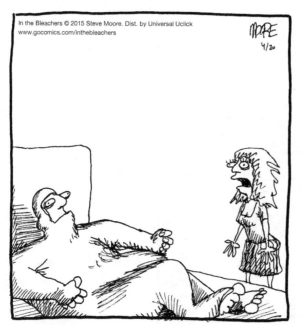

"It was a really bad idea to tell him
'Yoga rules, rugby drools' ..."

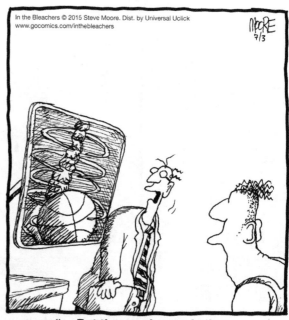

"... But the good news is that
you blocked his dunk!!"

In the Bleachers © 2014 Steve Moore. Dist. by Universal Uclick
www.gocomics.com/inthebleachers
MOORE
6/18

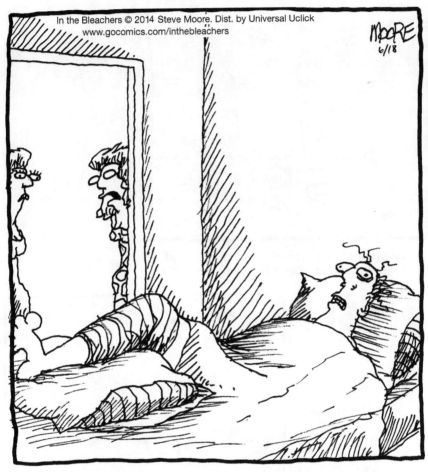

"The game is tied. Two outs in the ninth. Batter hits a high fly ball to the left. So Jason reaches for the TV remote to turn up the volume and tears the anterior cruciate ligament in his knee."

In the Bleachers © 2015 Steve Moore. Dist. by Universal Uclick
www.gocomics.com/inthebleachers 7/29
MOORE

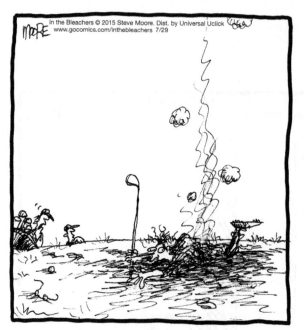

"Get up and tough it out! A real man would finish the round after a lightning strike!"

www.ucomics.com
© 2004 Universal Press Syndicate
MARATHON 103
MARATHON 204
MOORE
6·26

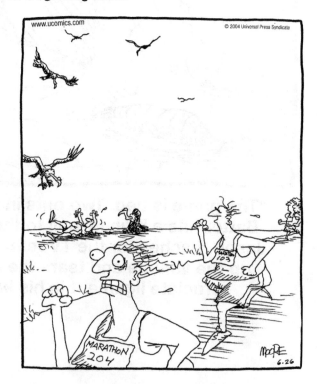

© 1996 Universal Press Syndicate
MOORE Jds Moore @ AOL.com
MARATHON
CLEANUP +
DISPOSAL
MARATHON
CLEANUP +
DISPOSAL
102
3-6

© 1999 Universal Press Syndicate
MOORE
12-29
www.uexpress.com

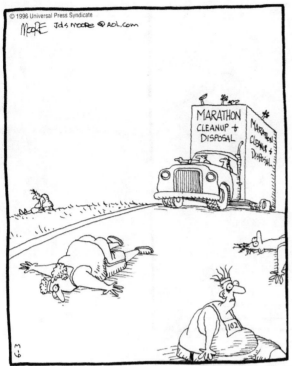

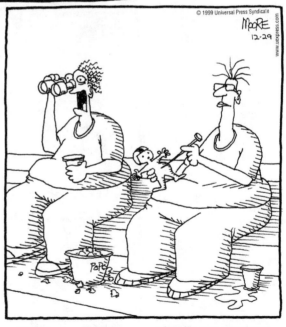

"This is so cool, Danny. ... Wait. The quarterback is trying to get back up. Stick him again! Stick him again!!"

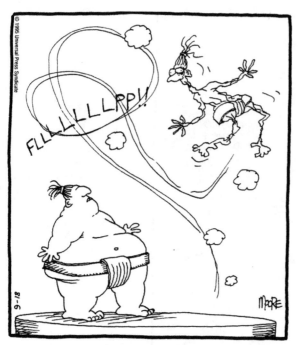

© 1995 Universal Press Syndicate
FLLLLLLLLPPP!!
9-18
MOORE

Sumo blowouts.

© 1995 Universal Press Syndicate
MOORE
9-25

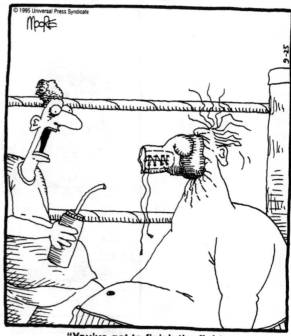

"You've got to finish the fight.
We can take X-rays later."

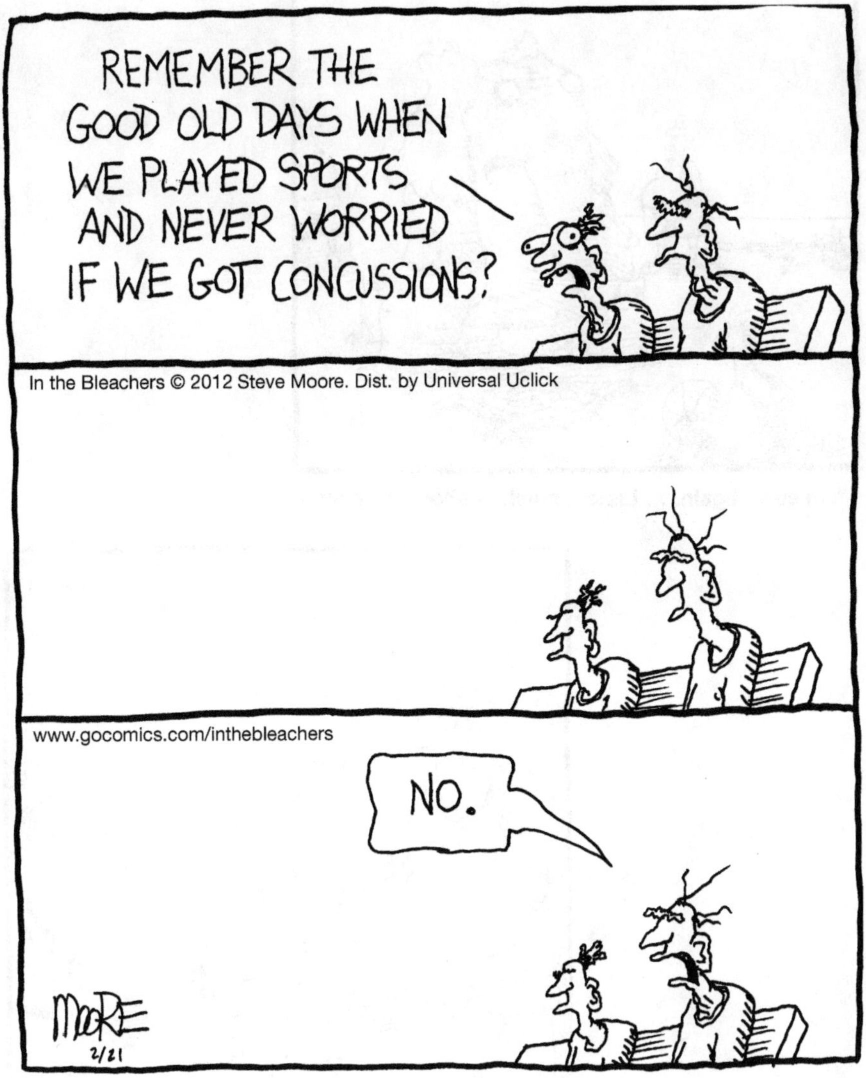
REMEMBER THE GOOD OLD DAYS WHEN WE PLAYED SPORTS AND NEVER WORRIED IF WE GOT CONCUSSIONS?
In the Bleachers © 2012 Steve Moore. Dist. by Universal Uclick
www.gocomics.com/inthebleachers
NO.
MOORE
2/21

© 1995 Universal Press Syndicate
MOORE

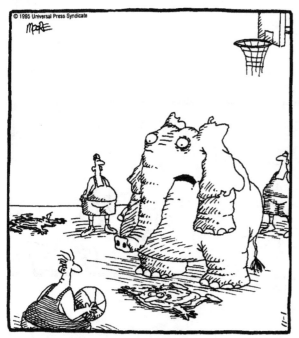

"I'm sorry again. ... Listen, maybe I shouldn't play."

© 1996 Universal Press Syndicate
MOORE

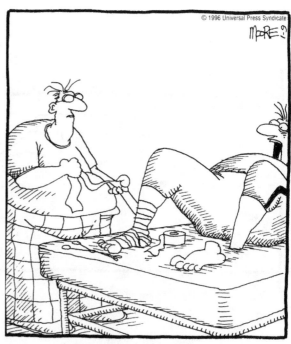

"Tape it up real tight, Floyd ... and the other ankle, too."

© 1998 Universal Press Syndicate
11-12
MOORE
www.uexpress.com

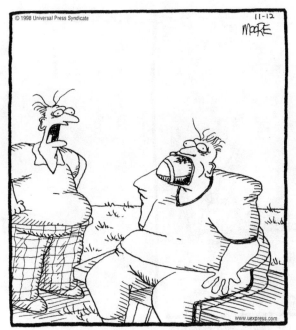

"It's really wedged in there. Well, I guess you'll remember to wear a mouth guard from now on."

© 1996 Universal Press Syndicate
SPLAT!!
MOORE
4-24

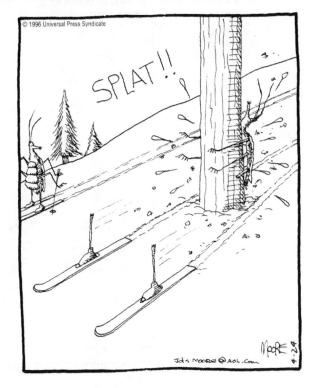

MOORE
9/15 In the Bleachers © 2015 Steve Moore. Dist. by Universal Uclick
www.gocomics.com/inthebleachers

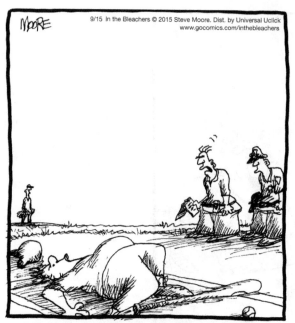

"We'll wait until CSI runs tests, but my gut feeling is that he was beaned in the head with some kind of hard, spherical object."

www.ucomics.com
© 2003 Universal Press Syndicate
MOORE
DOES IT HURT TO BEND IT?
11-17

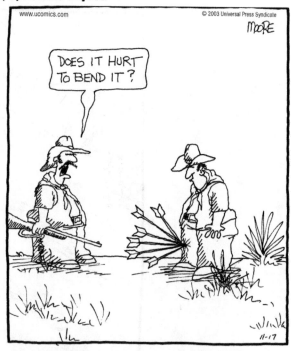

Career-ending knee injuries of the Wild West.

2-6
© 2004 Universal Press Syndicate
MOORE
SPOING!!
www.ucomics.com

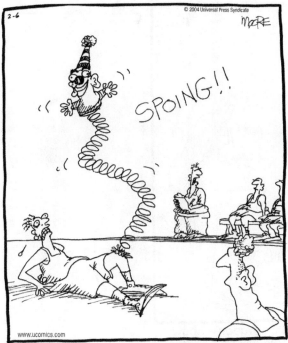

"McCarthy! Go in for Johnson. His knee popped out again."

© 2010 Universal Uclick www.gocomics.com
MOORE
5/15

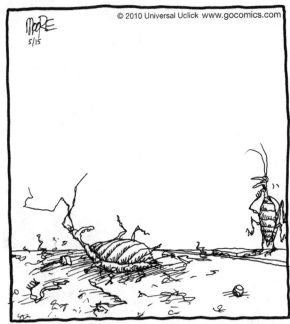

"Bad hop! Walk it off, babe, walk it off!!"

MOORE
www.ucomics.com
© 1997 Universal Press Syndicate 1-4

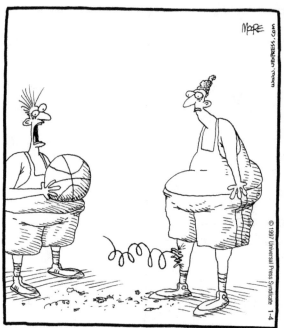

"Hey, I'm no orthopedic surgeon – know what I'm sayin'? But this can't be good."

© 2004 Universal Press Syndicate
11-5
MOORE
www.ucomics.com

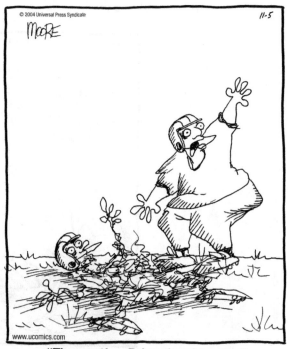

"Time out! ... Bring the air pump!"

www.ucomics.com
© 2004 Universal Press Syndicate
4-9
MOORE

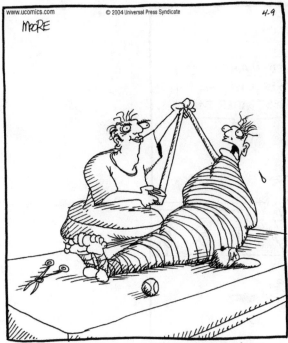

"Stop! That's enough! I just wanted my ankles taped!"

©2009 Universal Press Syndicate
www.gocomics.com
MOORE
2-23

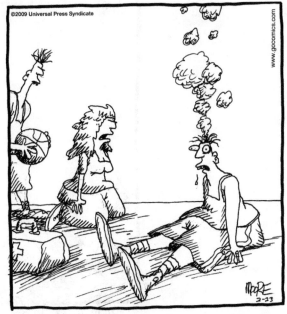

"I don't think it's a concussion ... although the smoke has me a little concerned."

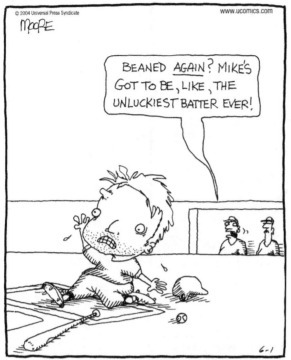

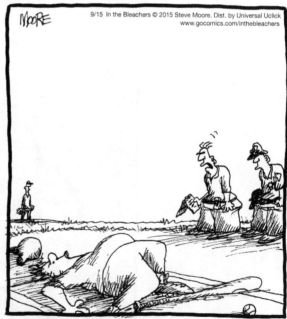

"We'll wait until CSI runs tests, but my gut feeling is that he was beaned in the head with some kind of hard, spherical object."

MOORE
5-27
www.gocomics.com
© 2009 Universal Press Syndicate

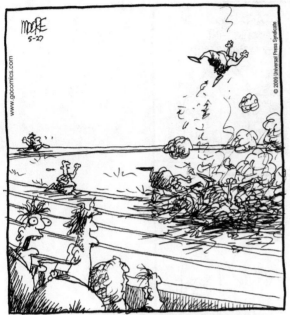

"I know it's sick, but I come to the track hoping to see accidents like this."

www.gocomics.com
MOORE
© 2006 Universal Press Syndicate
8-28

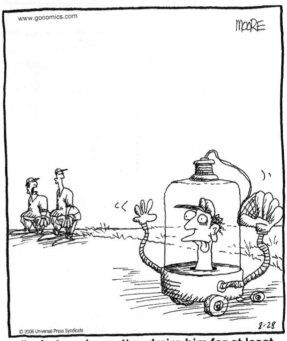

"... but you've gotta admire him for at least trying to come back after an injury of that magnitude."

GOLF? YEAH, I MISS THAT, TOO. AND I MISS SKIING.
AND SHOOTING HOOPS. AND SOFTBALL. AND...
MOORE
MAYBE WE SHOULDN'T TALK ABOUT SPORTS.
www.gocomics.com
© 2007 Universal Press Syndicate
6-25

www.gocomics.com
© 1996 Universal Press Syndicate
...WHEN I PLAYED FOOTBALL, WE DIDN'T WEAR HELMETS... WHEN I PLAYED FOOTBALL, WE DIDN'T WEAR HELMETS...WHEN I PLAYED FOOTBALL, WE...
MOORE
1/9

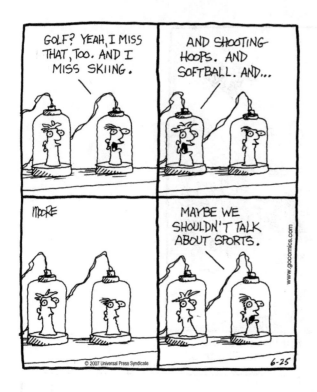

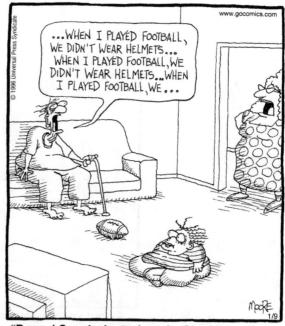

"Dewey! Grandpa's stuck again. Give him a couple of whacks upside the head."

© 2001 Universal Press Syndicate
MOORE
www.ucomics.com
1-23

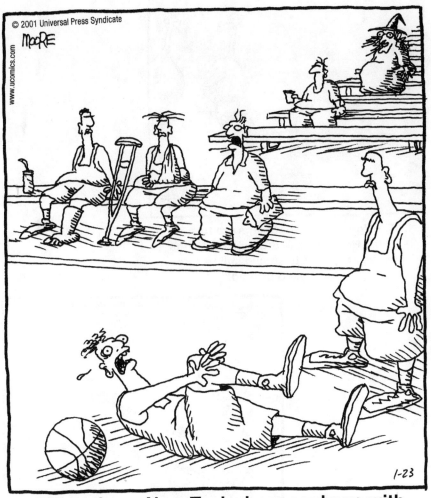

"What the ... Now Taylor's gone down with a career-ending injury. It's like we're cursed or something."

©2009 Universal Press Syndicate
www.gocomics.com
MOORE
3-13

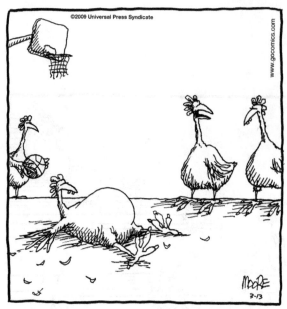

"The ligaments in both legs are torn to shreds. However, the drumsticks, thighs, wings and breasts should still be fine... either baked or fried."

© 2010 Universal Uclick www.gocomics.com
MOORE
7/13

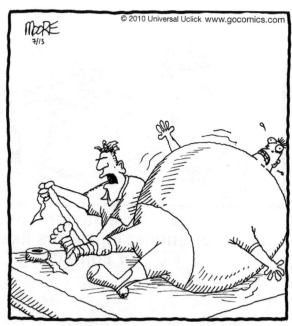

"I'm wrapping it tightly to keep the ankle from swelling."

© 2010 Universal Uclick www.gocomics.com
MOORE
3/30

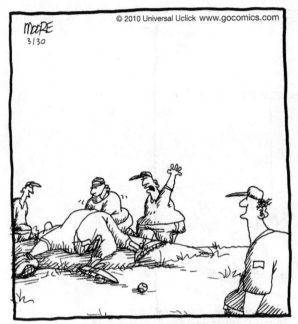

"Give us another minute, blue.
The surgeon just reattached the
tendon and he's closing up."

In the Bleachers © 2010 Steve Moore. Dist. by Universal Uclick
KNEE JOINT
REPLACEMENT
UNIT
MOORE
11/22

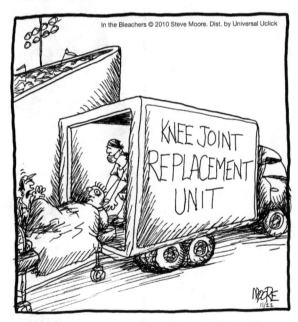

"This is a rush case ... Coach needs him
back for the fourth quarter."

© 2010 Universal Uclick www.gocomics.com
MOORE
6/26

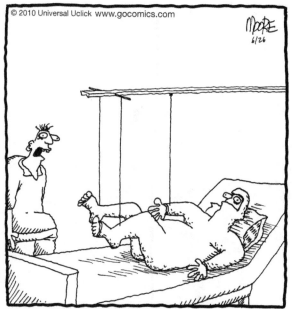

"Highlight reel on ESPN SportsCenter and ten million hits on YouTube ... Dude, you're *famous*!"

SLAM!!
In the Bleachers © 2010 Steve Moore. Dist. by Universal Uclick
MOORE
12/11

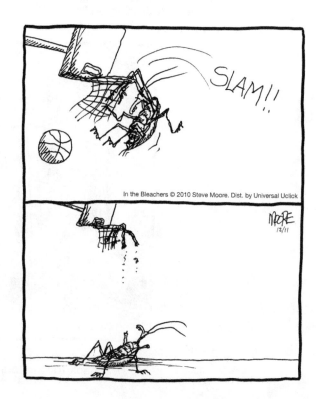

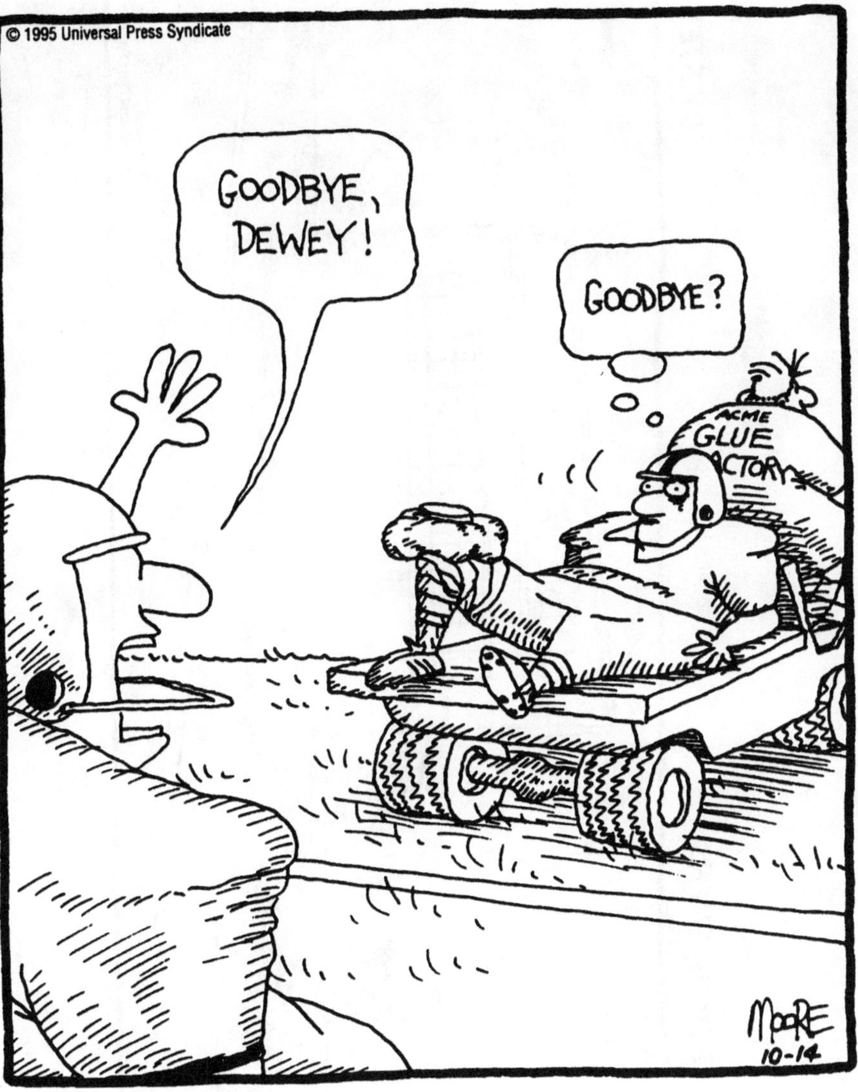
© 1995 Universal Press Syndicate
GOODBYE, DEWEY!
GOODBYE?
ACME GLUE FACTORY
MOORE 10-14

IN THE BLEACHERS

BY STEVE MOORE

www.ucomics.com
MOORE
LUBE AND TUNE
© 2003 Universal Press Syndicate
9-21

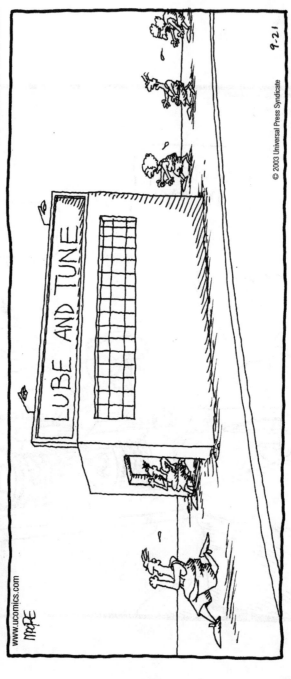

© 2010 Universal Uclick www.gocomics.com
MOORE
7/31

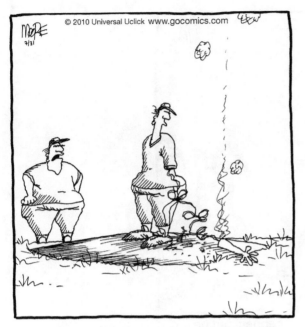

" ... 'Warm up before you take the mound,' I said. 'Stretch out,' I said. 'Loosen up,' I said ... Well, live and learn."

In the Bleachers © 2014 Steve Moore. Dist. by Universal Uclick
www.gocomics.com/inthebleachers
MOORE
7/16
PULLED HAMSTRINGS. TORN LIGAMENTS. BROKEN BONES... WHAT A MESS!

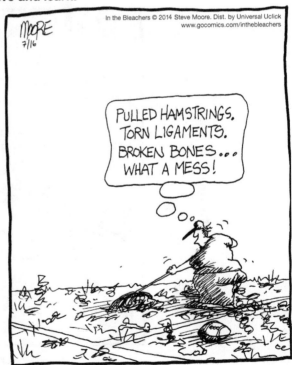

In the Bleachers © 2014 Steve Moore. Dist. by Universal Uclick
www.gocomics.com/inthebleachers
MOORE
3/15

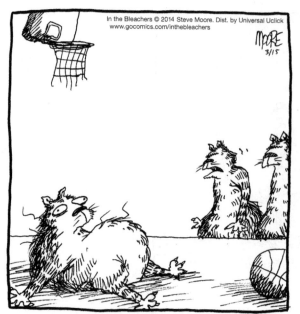

"I've never seen this happen, but he got injured when he grabbed the rebound and landed awkwardly on all four feet."

$5 ELBOW $5
RIGHT IN THE TEETH!!
MOORE
1-8
© 1998 Universal Press Syndicate www.uexpress.com
JdSmooRe @ AoL.Com

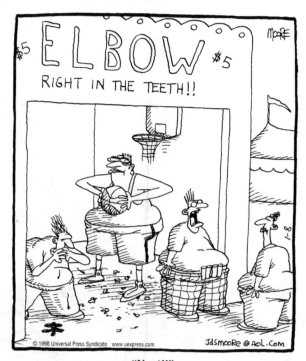

"Next!!"

MARATHON
FINISH
FINISHER
MOORE
© 2003 Universal Press Syndicate
www.ucomics.com
6.20

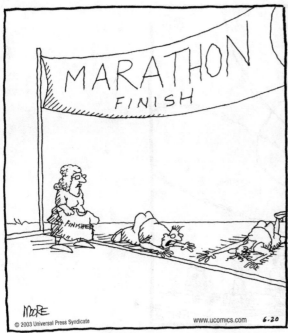

"Wait. ... Forget the T-shirt. It's reeeeal close, but his hand's not quite over the line."

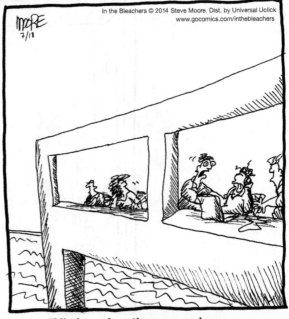

In the Bleachers © 2014 Steve Moore. Dist. by Universal Uclick
www.gocomics.com/inthebleachers
MOORE
7/18

"His broadcasting career is over. He tore ligaments in his tongue!"

www.gocomics.com/inthebleachers
MOORE 8/7
In the Bleachers © 2014 Steve Moore. Dist. by Universal Uclick

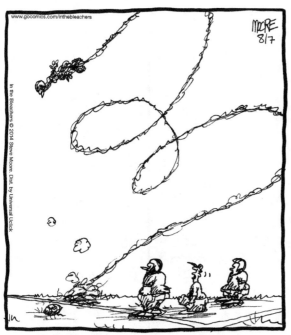

"He'll be OK. He just got the wind knocked out of him."

www.uexpress.com
© 2000 Universal Press Syndicate
MOORE 9-8

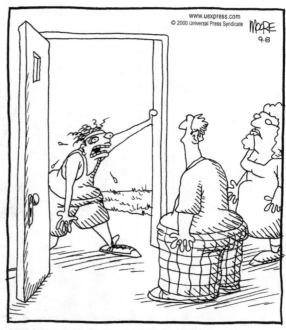

"Hi. Can I use your phone? I was jogging past your house and my cardiovascular system broke down."

In the Bleachers © 2014 Steve Moore. Dist. by Universal Uclick
www.gocomics.com/inthebleachers
MOORE
9/8

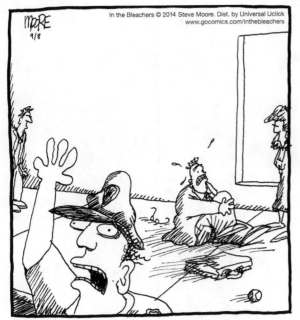

"Move along! Move along! I'm sure you've all seen a guy hit by a line drive right in the shin before!!"

In the Bleachers © 2015 Steve Moore. Dist. by Universal Uclick
www.gocomics.com/inthebleachers
MOORE
2/7

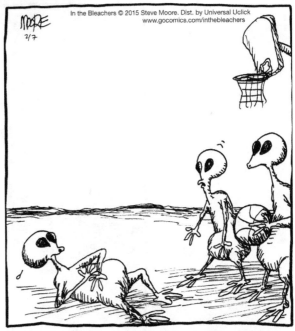

"He'll be OK. He just got the carbon dioxide, argon and nitrogen knocked out of him."

In the Bleachers © 2014 Steve Moore. Dist. by Universal Uclick
www.gocomics.com/inthebleachers
MOORE
8/28
70

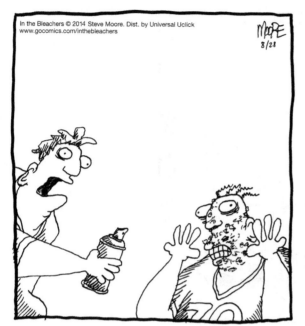

"Try this, Bryan. It's guaranteed to cure athlete's face on contact!"

MOORE
10/16
In the Bleachers © 2014 Steve Moore. Dist. by Universal Uclick
www.gocomics.com/inthebleachers
INJURED RESERVE
PLEASE DO NOT FEED THEIR HOPES

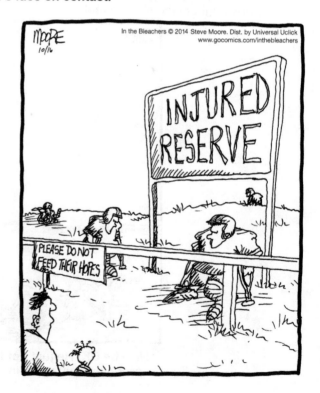

www.gocomics.com/inthebleachers
In the Bleachers © 2014 Steve Moore. Dist. by Universal Uclick
MOORE
10/21
WHERE DOES IT HURT?
HOME FOR RETIRED ATHLETIC TRAINERS

In the Bleachers © 2015 Steve Moore. Dist. by Universal Uclick
www.gocomics.com/inthebleachers
MOORE
1/27
WILL RUPTURE SPLEENS FOR ANOTHER CHANCE IN THE NFL

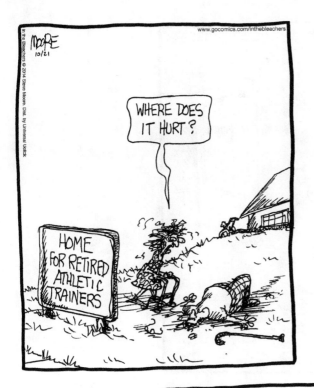

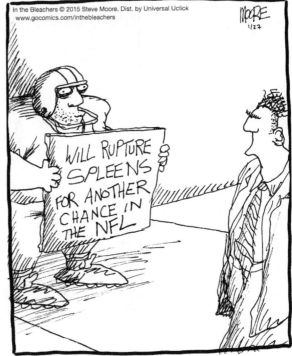

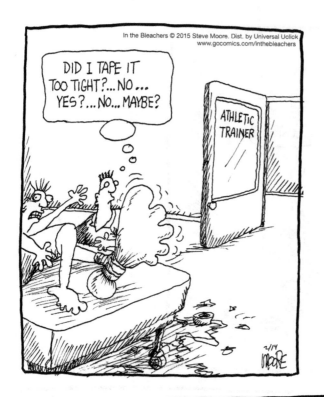

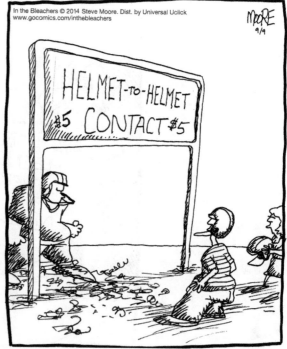

In the Bleachers © 2014 Steve Moore. Dist. by Universal Uclick
www.gocomics.com/inthebleachers
MOORE
12/8

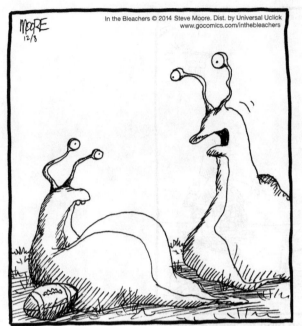

"Well, you're lucky. You don't seem to have any broken bones. HA! ... Sorry. Anyhoo ..."

In the Bleachers © 2015 Steve Moore. Dist. by Universal Uclick 8/7
www.gocomics.com/inthebleachers
MOORE
I HELD ONTO THE BALL!!
GO GET HELP.

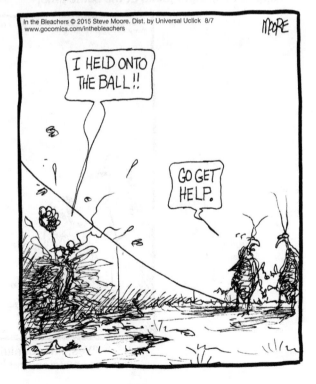

MOORE
3/13
In the Bleachers © 2015 Steve Moore. Dist. by Universal Uclick
www.gocomics.com/inthebleachers

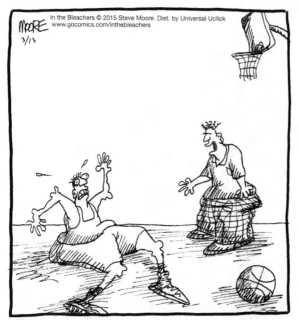

"This is so cool! I've seen elbows, wrists, knees and ankles blown out, but I've never seen it happen to all eight joints at the same time!"

In the Bleachers © 2015 Steve Moore. Dist. by Universal Uclick
www.gocomics.com/inthebleachers
MOORE
2/13

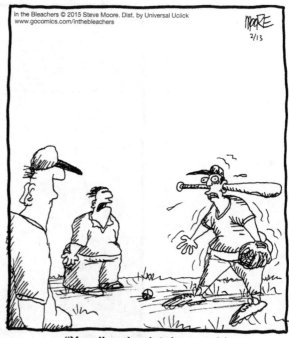

"Yes, I'm absolutely sure. It's a concussion and he cannot play."

© 1995 Universal Press Syndicate
MOORE

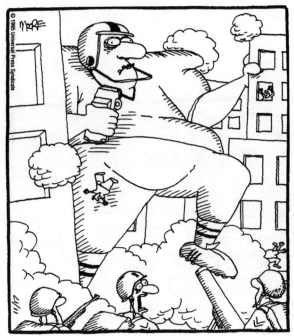

"Aim for his knee ligaments! It's our only hope!"

© 1995 Universal Press Syndicate
MOORE
9-20

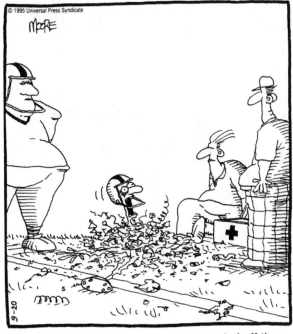

"Yo, Coach! Does this mean I get carried off the field on the back of that cool little golf cart?"

MOORE 7/22
In the Bleachers © 2015 Steve Moore. Dist. by Universal Uclick
www.gocomics.com/inthebleachers
ON THE SNAP, EVERYONE COLLAPSE ON THE GROUND, CLUTCHING YOUR KNEE, JUST TO MESS WITH COACH.

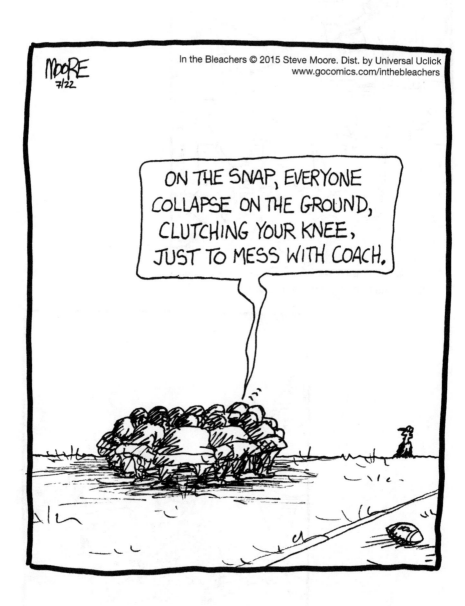

MOORE
8/27 In the Bleachers © 2015 Steve Moore. Dist. by Universal Uclick
www.gocomics.com/inthebleachers

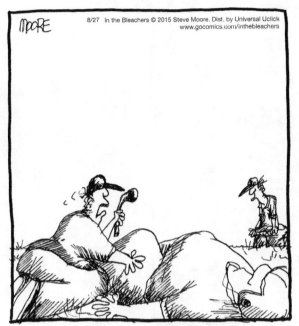

"Fool! I asked for a *knee* replacement. This is an artificial hip!!"

MOORE
In the Bleachers © 2015 Steve Moore. Dist. by Universal Uclick
www.gocomics.com/inthebleachers

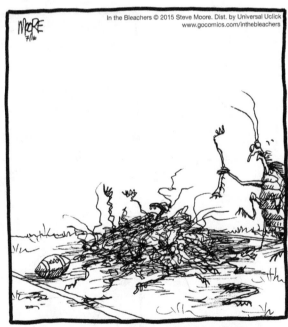

"No one move! Let's unfold this pile in an orderly manner ... So who's leg is this?"

In the Bleachers © 2015 Steve Moore. Dist. by Universal Uclick 10/8
www.gocomics.com/inthebleachers
MOORE

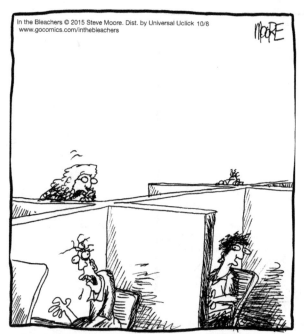

"It's fantasy football, Matthew. He's faking it. He cannot possibly have a concussion."

© 1996 Universal Press Syndicate
MOORE
YOU'VE GOT SLIVERS. TWO OF THEM. AND THEY'RE REALLY DEEP...
2-13

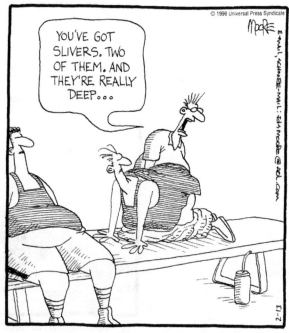

Benchwarmer with a career-ending injury.

HE JUST GOT THE WIND KNOCKED OUT OF HIM.
MOORE 4/8
OK. MAYBE HE'S DEAD.

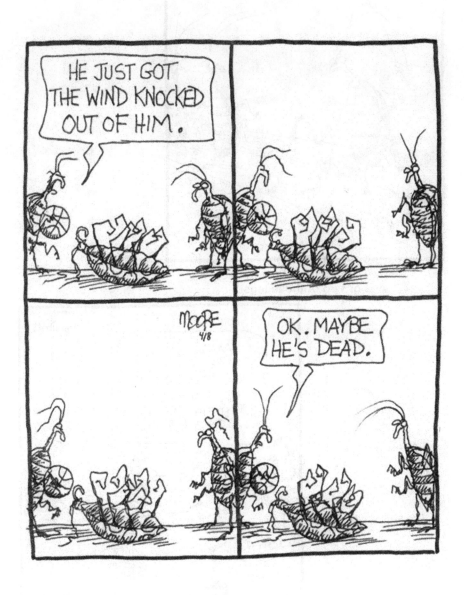

In the Bleachers © 2015 Steve Moore. Dist. by Universal Uclick 8/17
www.gocomics.com/inthebleachers
MOORE

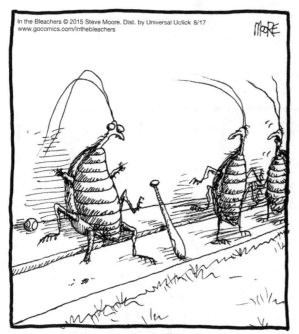

"Dewey's out until he grows back one or two of those legs."

© 1995 Universal Press Syndicate
MOORE
AAAAAAH!! I TORE MY ANTERIOR CRUCIATE LIGAMENT INTO A BILLION TINY PIECES!! ... JUST KIDDING.
10-24

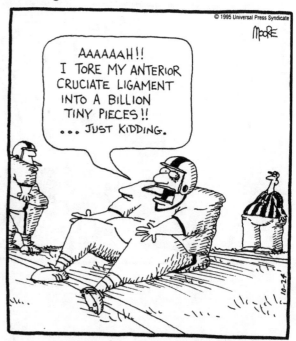

And then, one day, Andy's career really did come to an end, but no one believed him.

© 1996 Universal Press Syndicate
MOORE
FACIALS
$5
3-7

www.uexpress.com
© 1999 Universal Press Syndicate
MOORE
9-10
IN CASE OF INJURIES, BREAK GLASS

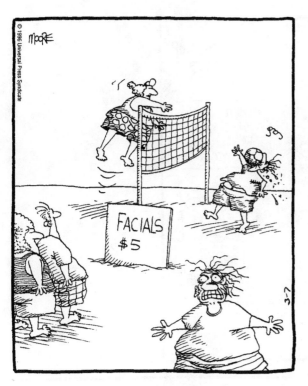

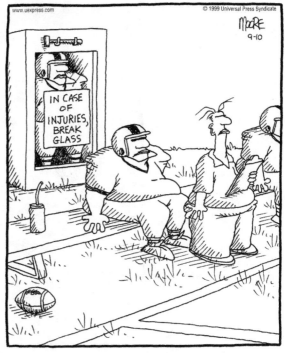

LAST WEEK I FOUND A DEFENSIVE BACK WITH A PULLED GROIN BUT IN OTHERWISE PERFECT CONDITION.
OOOH, LOOK! A PLACE-KICKER! I WONDER IF HE'S STILL ACCURATE.
STADIUM DISPOSAL INC.
MOORE 11-12
www.uexpress.com
© 1999 Universal Press Syndicate

MOORE
3-29
© 1996 Universal Press Syndicate

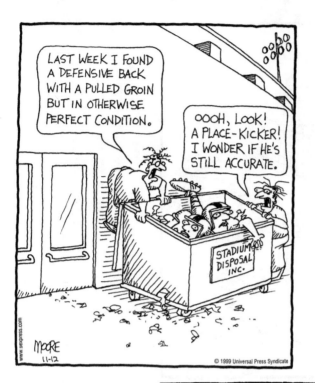

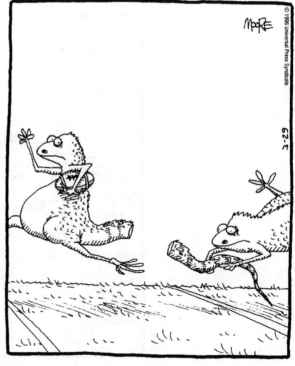

YOU BROKE YOUR LEG. I'LL TAPE YOU UP AND GET YOU BACK IN THE GAME.
© 1999 Universal Press Syndicate
3-16
MOORE
www.uexpress.com
YOU BROKE EVERY BONE IN YOUR BODY. I'LL TAPE YOU UP AND GET YOU BACK IN THE GAME.

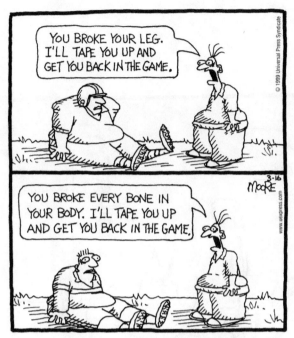

The difference between football and rugby.

11/18
MOORE
© 1995 Universal Press Syndicate

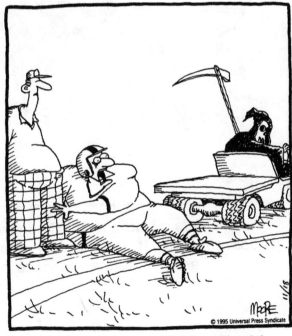

"No! Don't make me go! I'll play with pain! I'll play with pain!"

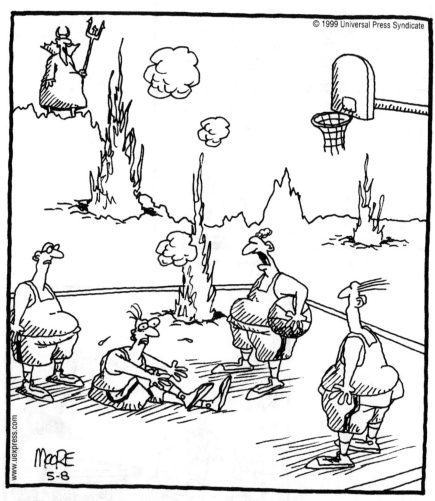

© 1999 Universal Press Syndicate

www.uexpress.com

MOORE
5-8

"Whoa. That's a bad sprain. Ordinarily, I'd tell you to put some ice on it, but your chances of finding any around here are slim to none."

© 1998 Universal Press Syndicate
8-14 MOORE
WITH A THIRD-BASE COACH
WHAM!!
WITHOUT A THIRD-BASE COACH
www.uexpress.com

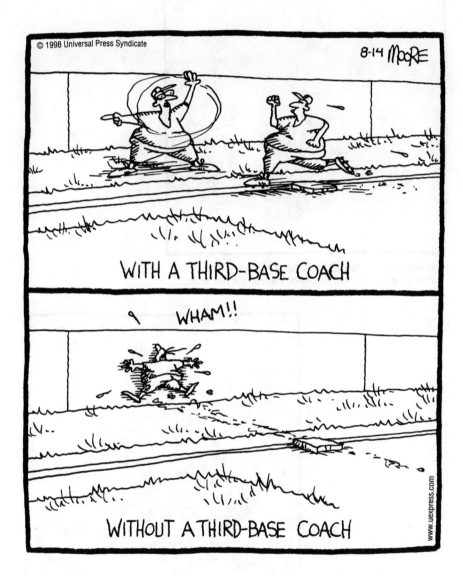

E-MAIL, SCHMEE-MAIL: JdsMOORE @AOL.COM
MOORE
© 1996 Universal Press Syndicate
2-17

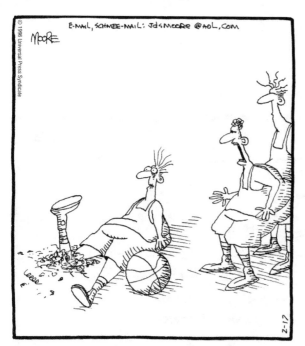

"Where do you hurt? Your back? Ankle? Shoulder? Neck? Knee? ... He blinked! I think it's his knee."

JdsMOORE @AOL.COM
© 1996 Universal Press Syndicate
...AND CARL MAKES A GRUNTING NOISE WHEN HE SWINGS.
OH, OK. LET'S TALK ABOUT ANNOYING SOUNDS, MR. CHRONIC STOMACH GAS!
THEY NEVER LET ME DRIVE THE CART.
PLEASE STOP YELLING!!
KLEENEX
9-16 MOORE

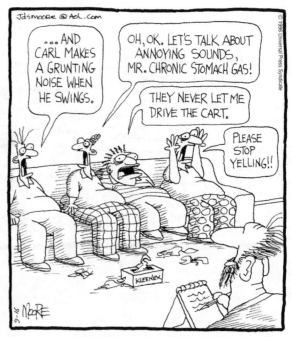

Golf foursome in counseling.

© 2003 Universal Press Syndicate
MOORE
www.ucomics.com
3-4

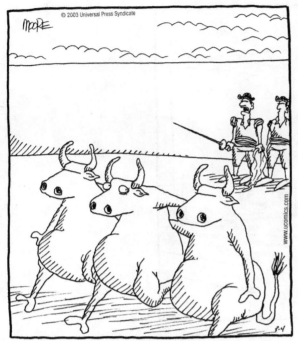

"Wait a minute. How do we know he's not just *faking* a knee injury?"

MOORE
© 1999 Universal Press Syndicate
4-21
www.uexpress.com

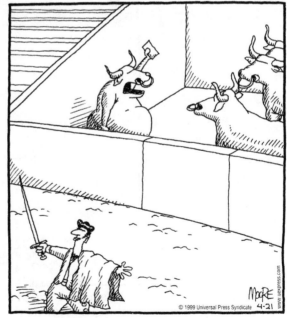

"OK, before the fights begin, has everyone completely filled out his organ-donor card?"

© 1999 Universal Press Syndicate
www.uexpress.com
FISH FOOD
MOORE 10-21

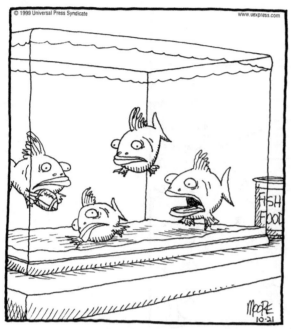

"If it's a torn ligament, we might as well flush him down the toilet."

© 2001 Universal Press Syndicate
www.ucomics.com
MOORE
104
211
167
79
1-16

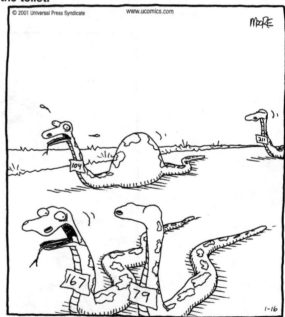

"It's her own fault. She can't just squeeze a pig to death and swallow it whole right before a marathon, and not expect to get stomach cramps."

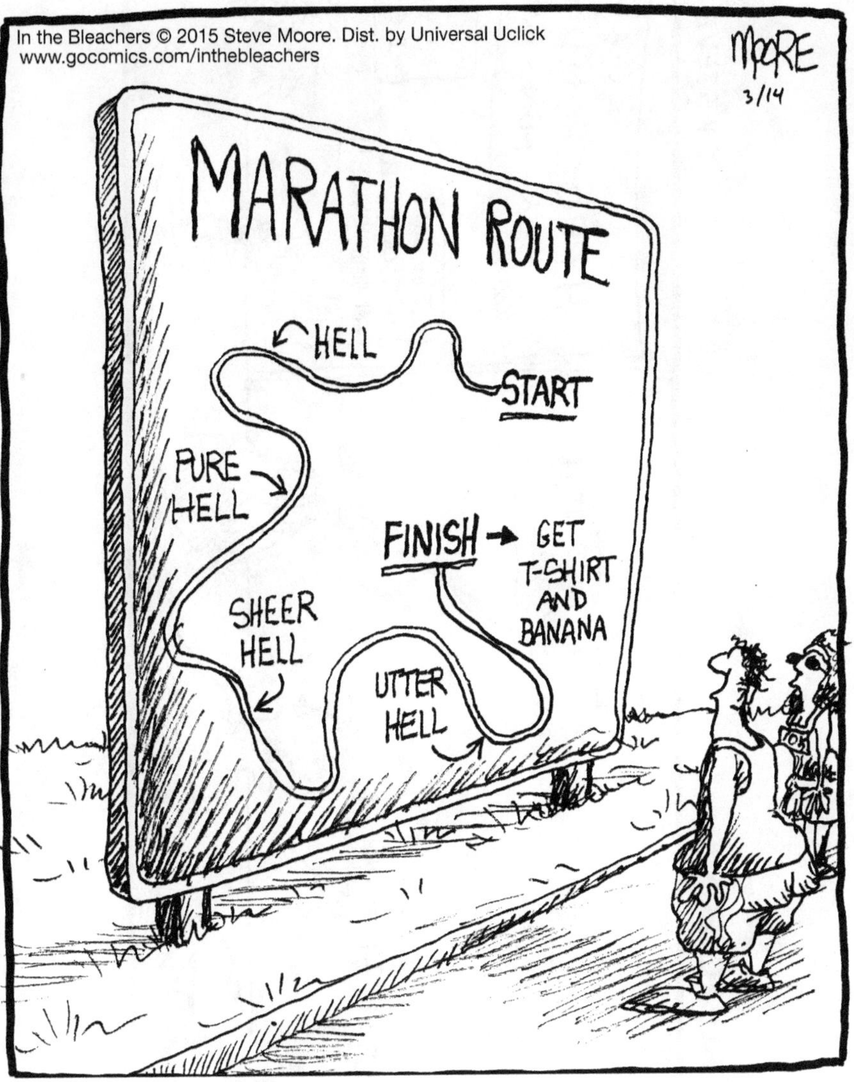
In the Bleachers © 2015 Steve Moore. Dist. by Universal Uclick
www.gocomics.com/inthebleachers
MOORE
3/14
MARATHON ROUTE
HELL
START
PURE HELL
FINISH
GET T-SHIRT AND BANANA
SHEER HELL
UTTER HELL

IN THE BLEACHERS BY STEVE MOORE

www.ucomics.com
MOORE
© 2001 Universal Press Syndicate
YOU LOOK AS BAD AS I FEEL.
I KNEW IT! I'M DYING!!
MY KNEE HURTS. IT'S PROBABLY RABIES!
ANNUAL HYPOCHONDRIAC 10K FUN RUN
I'VE GOT A SIDEACHE—CALL AN AMBULANCE!
THERE GO MY SINUSES. I QUIT.
12/21

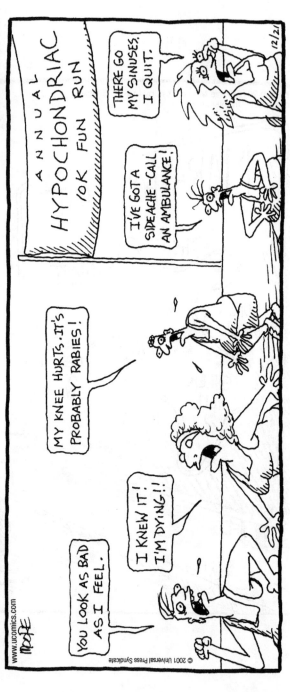

In the Bleachers © 2011 Steve Moore. Dist. by Universal Uclick
MOORE
10/19
ATHLETIC
TRAINER

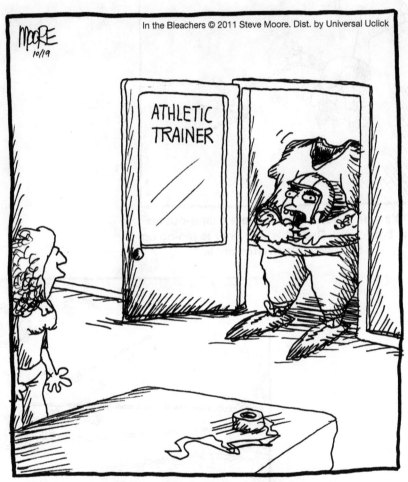

"Can you tape me up?"

©2009 Universal Press Syndicate
MOORE
2-13
www.gocomics.com

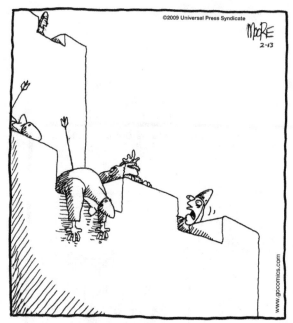

"It's safe to look, sire. There's a time-out on the battlefield. Our athletic trainer is taping up Sir Dwayne's twisted ankle."

© 2009 Universal Press Syndicate
www.gocomics.com
MOORE
5-2

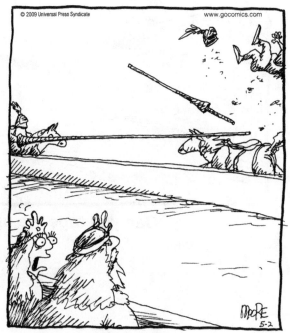

"Size matters!"

© 2006 Universal Press Syndicate
CHICKA-TUK!
CHICKA-TUK!
CHICKA-TUK!
CONCUSSION BE-GONE
INTHEBLEACHERS.COM
MOORE
12-2 www.gocomics.com

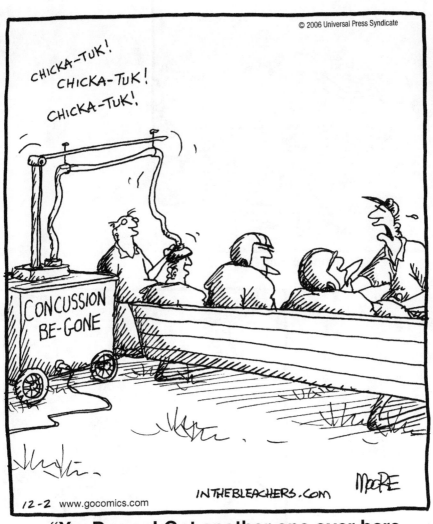

"Yo, Dewey! Got another one over here when you're done."

© 2007 Universal Press Syndicate
MOORE
www.gocomics.com
3-16

"Someone should fix that."

© 2007 Universal Press Syndicate
3-12
MOORE
www.gocomics.com

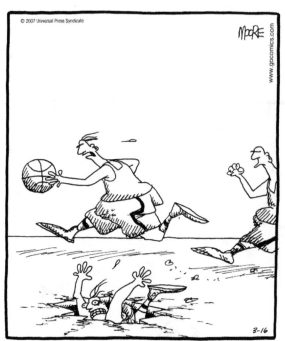

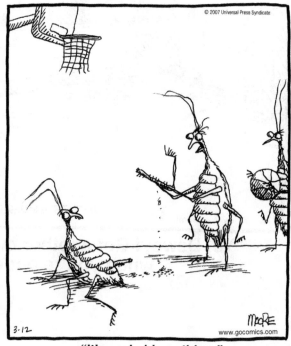

"It's probably nothing."

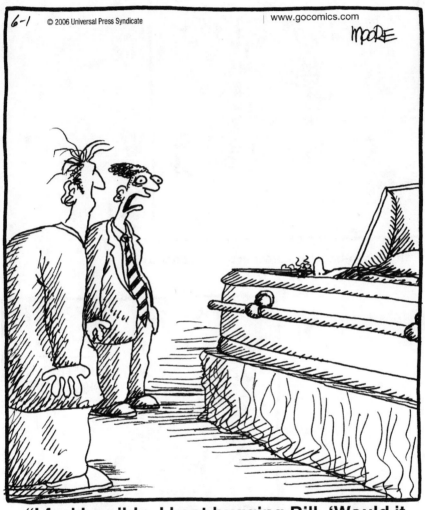

6-1
© 2006 Universal Press Syndicate
www.gocomics.com
MOORE

"I feel horrible. I kept bugging Bill, 'Would it kill you to pass me the ball? Huh? Would it?' ... And then, in the fourth quarter, Bill finally passed me the ball."

© 2007 Universal Press Syndicate
WAAAAAAH!!
DAYCAR
11-12
www.gocomics.com
MOORE

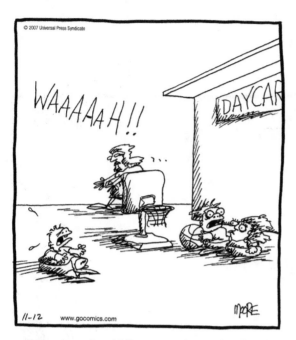

"It's a boo-boo! His career in professional sports is over!"

www.gocomics.com
ME HOPE GORK WEARING A CUP.
© 2009 Universal Press Syndicate
MOORE
8-8

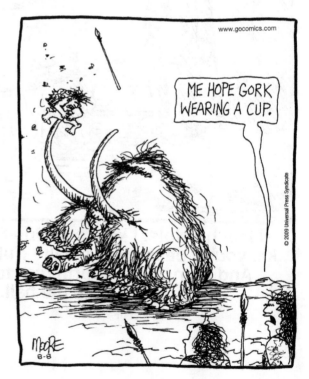

© 2000 Universal Press Syndicate
www.uexpress.com
MOORE
4-27

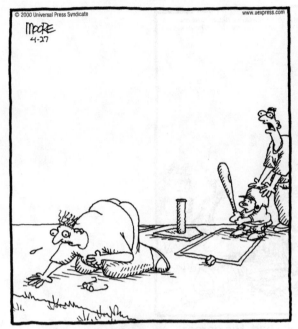

"Good contact, Tristin. Very, very nice. But next time, wait until your coach sets the ball on the tee before you swing."

THE CENTER FIELDER IS GOING BACK—WAAAAY BACK—TO A HORRIBLE MEMORY THAT'S BEEN REPRESSED FOR MANY YEARS!
© 2000 Universal Press Syndicate
www.uexpress.com
MOORE
8-26

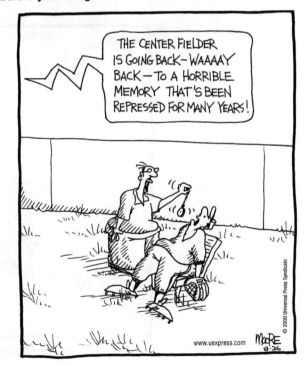

MOORE
9/19 In the Bleachers © 2016 Steve Moore. Dist. by Universal Uclick
www.gocomics.com/inthebleachers

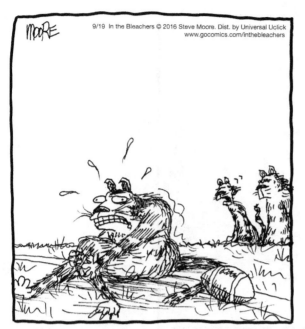

"It's bad, coach. Really bad. His career is over ... All nine of them."

MOORE
7/15
In the Bleachers © 2013 Steve Moore. Dist. by Universal Uclick
www.gocomics.com/inthebleachers

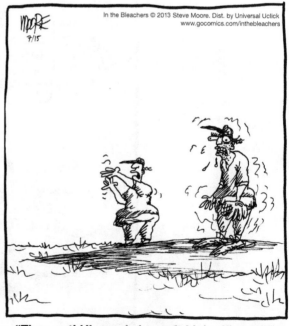

"Time out! His meds haven't kicked in yet!!"

www.ucomics.com
© 2002 Universal Press Syndicate
MOORE
TRUST ME, BOYS. YOU MAY HATE ME NOW, BUT ONE DAY WHEN THE WOUNDS HAVE HEALED YOU'LL THANK ME FOR HOLDING SLIDING PRACTICE ON AN ASPHALT PARKING LOT.
6·6

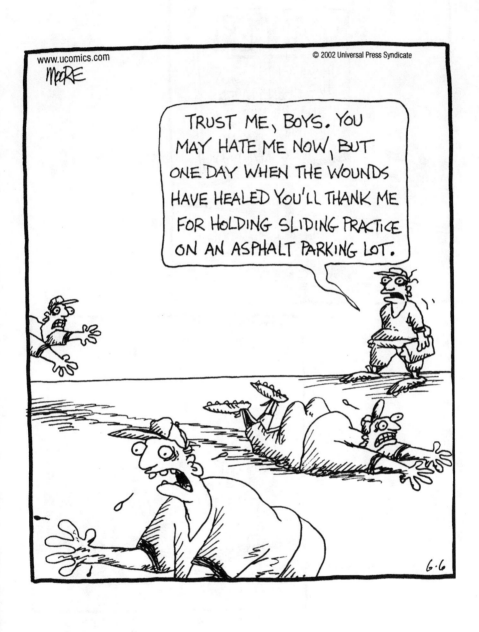

In the Bleachers © 2011 Steve Moore. Dist. by Universal Uclick
MOORE 9/16
DANGER!
THIS WARNING SIGN HAS BEEN PLACED RIGHT IN THE MIDDLE OF THE TRACK FOR NO APPARENT REASON!

© 2009 Universal Press Syndicate
MOORE 6-6
www.gocomics.com

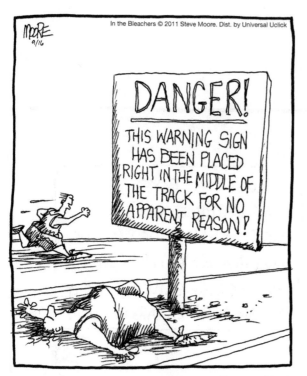

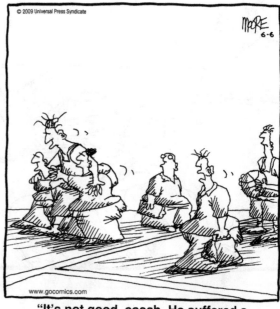

"It's not good, coach. He suffered a traumatic blow to his ego. I can't promise anything, but with intense psychotherapy he might be back in 10 years."

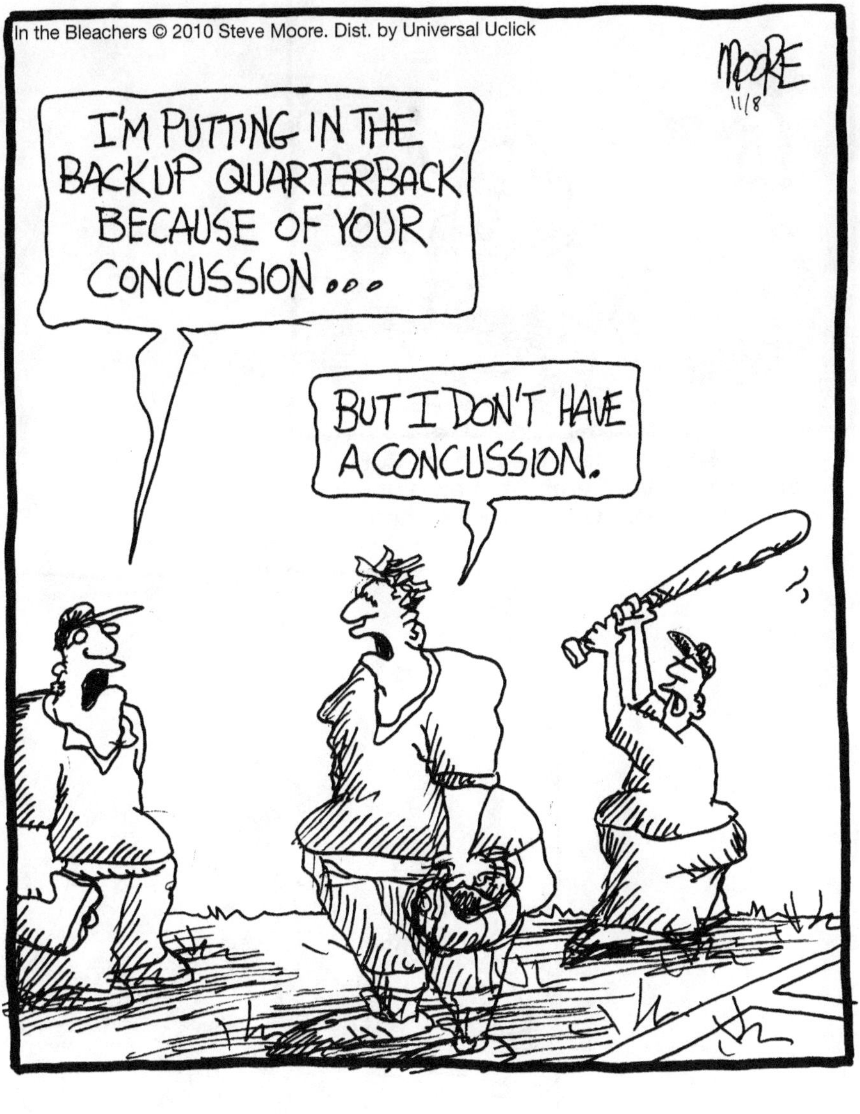
MOORE 11/8
I'M PUTTING IN THE BACKUP QUARTERBACK BECAUSE OF YOUR CONCUSSION...
BUT I DON'T HAVE A CONCUSSION.

© 2009 Universal Press Syndicate
MOORE
9-11
www.gocomics.com

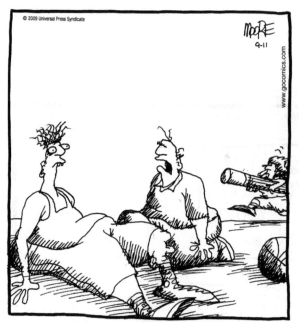

"Your knee is totally messed up. But don't worry. We'll erase it, draw a new one and get you back in the game."

MOORE
9-1
© 2009 Universal Press Syndicate
www.gocomics.com

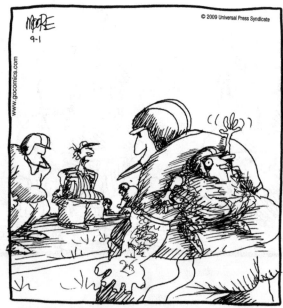

"Nothing? Well, keep looking! A quarterback doesn't go down under a pile of tacklers and just vanish from the face of the Earth."

© 2009 Universal Press Syndicate
www.gocomics.com
MOORE
7-24
BOB'S
ARM FIX

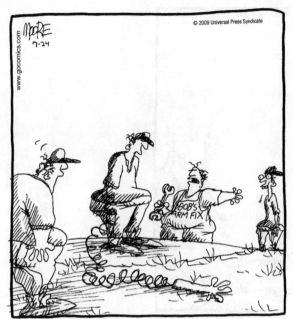

"It'll take a day or two to get the parts. Meanwhile, here's a loaner."

In the Bleachers © 2016 Steve Moore. Dist. by Universal Uclick 2/4
www.gocomics.com/inthebleachers
MOORE

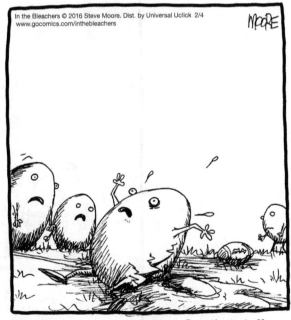

"That's not just a fracture. See that stuff leaking out? It's a compound fracture!"

In the Bleachers © 2013 Steve Moore. Dist. by Universal Uclick
www.gocomics.com/inthebleachers
MOORE 6/20

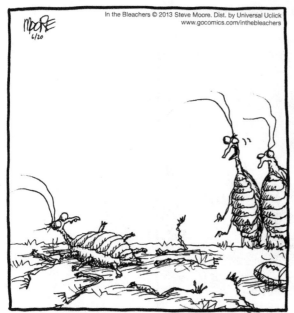

"I'll know more when I see X-rays, but my guess is that he got ripped apart, limb by limb."

© 2009 Universal Press Syndicate
MOORE 8-19
www.gocomics.com
TIME OUT!!

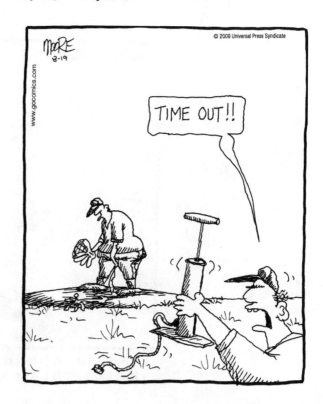

In the Bleachers © 2013 Steve Moore. Dist. by Universal Uclick
www.gocomics.com/inthebleachers
MOORE
6/18

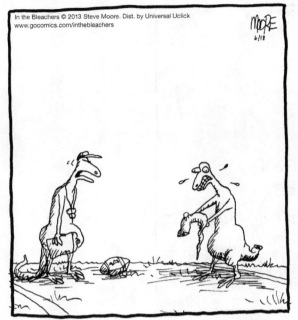

"Don't come whining to me. Go see the athletic trainer and get it taped up."

In the Bleachers © 2013 Steve Moore. Dist. by Universal Uclick
www.gocomics.com/inthebleachers
MOORE
7/18

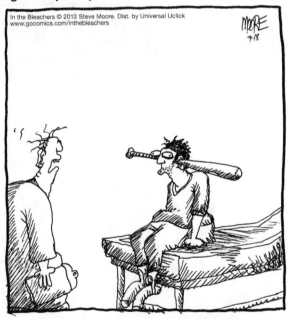

"Yes. I can remove it at great risk and expense. Or ... we leave it in and you are blessed for the rest of your life with an excellent conversation starter."

© 2010 Universal Uclick www.gocomics.com
MOORE 9/14

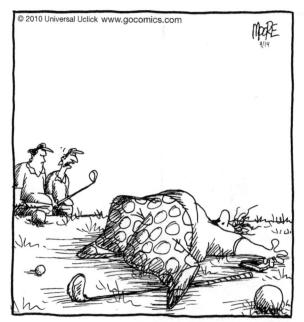

"I warned him. 'Don't text and drive' ... He wouldn't listen."

© 2010 Universal Uclick www.gocomics.com
LOOK UP... LOOK DOWN... LOOK AT MY THUMB. GEE, YOU'RE...
QUIT MESSING AROUND, DOC! DOES HE HAVE A CONCUSSION OR NOT?
MOORE 9/15

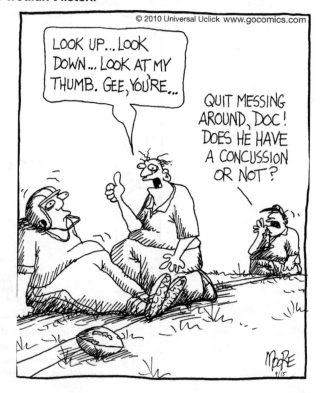

© 2009 Universal Uclick
www.gocomics.com
MOORE
11-12
SHUT UP!
YOU SHUT UP!!
HIS BAD KNEE IS ACTING UP AGAIN.

© 2010 Universal Uclick www.gocomics.com
MOORE
3-23
HE HELD ONTO THE BALL!!

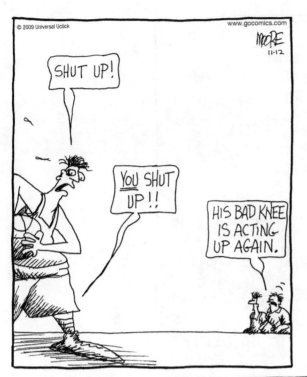

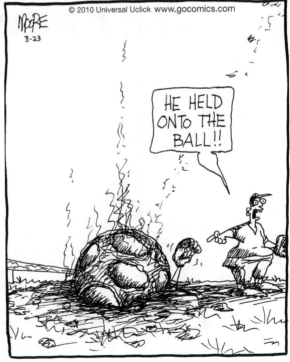

© 2009 Universal Uclick
www.gocomics.com
MOORE 11-21
WELL, THIS IS YOUR LUCKY DAY, SHEEDY. GO IN FOR MOORE... HE JUST BLEW OUT HIS KNEE.

© 2010 Universal Uclick www.gocomics.com
LEGO
MOORE

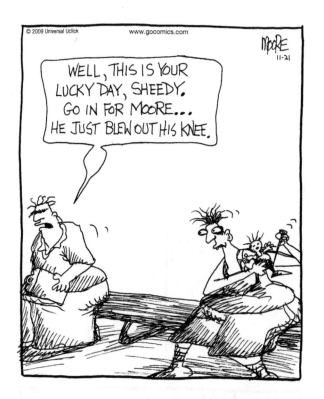

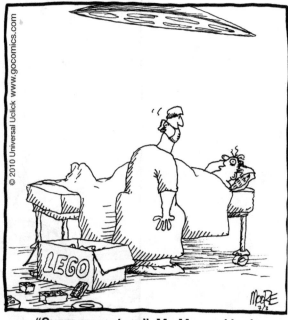

"Surgery went well, Mr. Moore. I had a lot of fun rebuilding your knee joint."

© 2009 Universal Uclick
www.gocomics.com

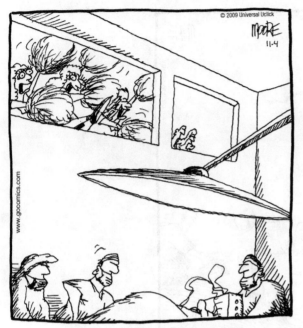

"L-I-G-A-M-E-N-T!" Ligament!
Ligament! Yee-aaaaay, ligament!"

© 2010 Universal Uclick www.gocomics.com

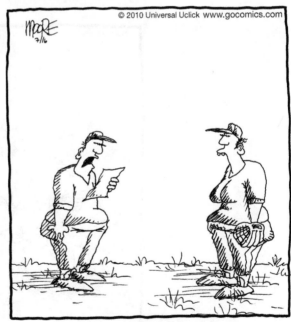

"Good news and bad news, Kevin.
You tested negative for steroids,
but positive for estrogen."

© 2009 Universal Uclick
MOORE
10-5
www.gocomics.com

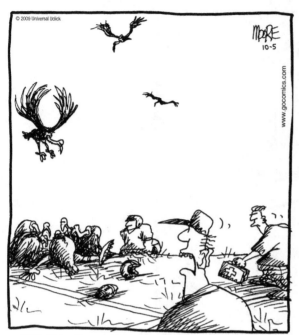

"Wait! Let's see if he gets up on his own."

© 2009 Universal Uclick
www.gocomics.com
MOORE
12-17

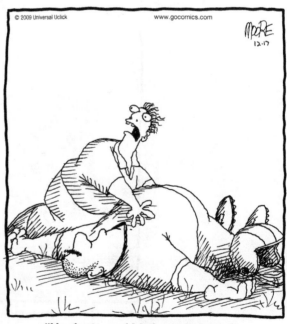

"He destroyed his inner balance! ...
Get the yoga coach!"

© 2002 Universal Press Syndicate
www.ucomics.com
MOORE
8-9

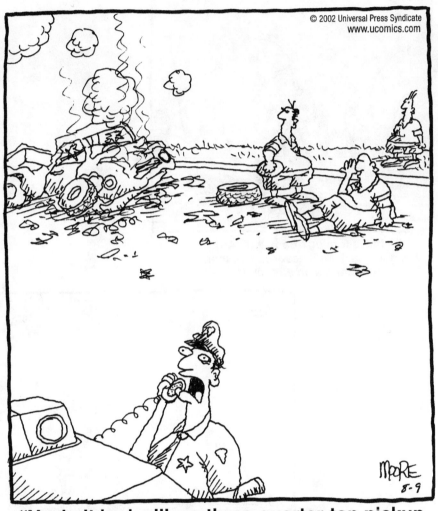

"Yeah, it looks like a three-quarter-ton pickup truck collided head-on with a rugby player. ... What's that? ... Oh, yeah. It's totaled."

© 2010 Universal Uclick www.gocomics.com
MOORE
3-13

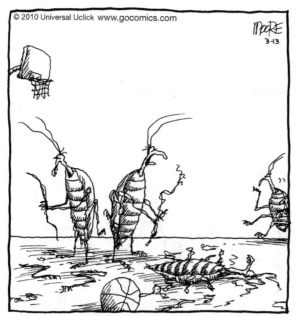

"Is this a foreleg? Back leg? Antenna? It's hopeless! We'll never ... Oh, thank God. Here comes an athletic trainer!"

In the Bleachers © 2011 Steve Moore. Dist. by Universal Uclick
MOORE
2/23

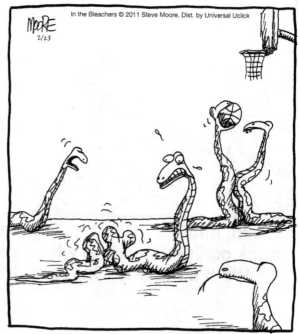

"It's just a cramp, Vince! Slither it off, babe! Slither it off!!"

MOORE
www.gocomics.com
© 2006 Universal Press Syndicate
8-29

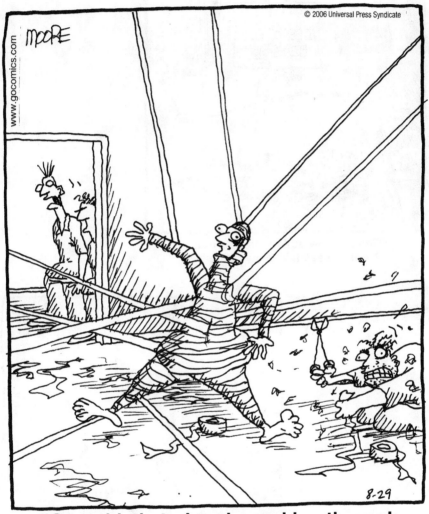

"Our athletic trainer is working through some 'issues' ..."

In the Bleachers © 2011 Steve Moore. Dist. by Universal Uclick
MOORE 3/15
DOES THIS TICKLE? WHAT ABOUT THIS?...
YES! YES! I BEG OF YOU! PLEASE STOP!!

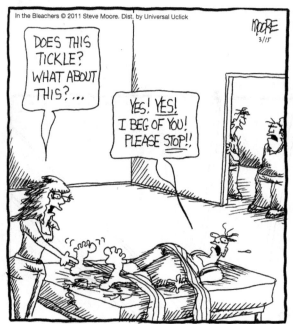

"Tell the new athletic trainer that I want to see her in my office."

In the Bleachers © 2011 Steve Moore. Dist. by Universal Uclick
MOORE 3/17

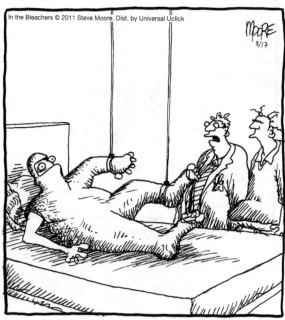

"He's a lucky man, coach. His throwing arm is OK."

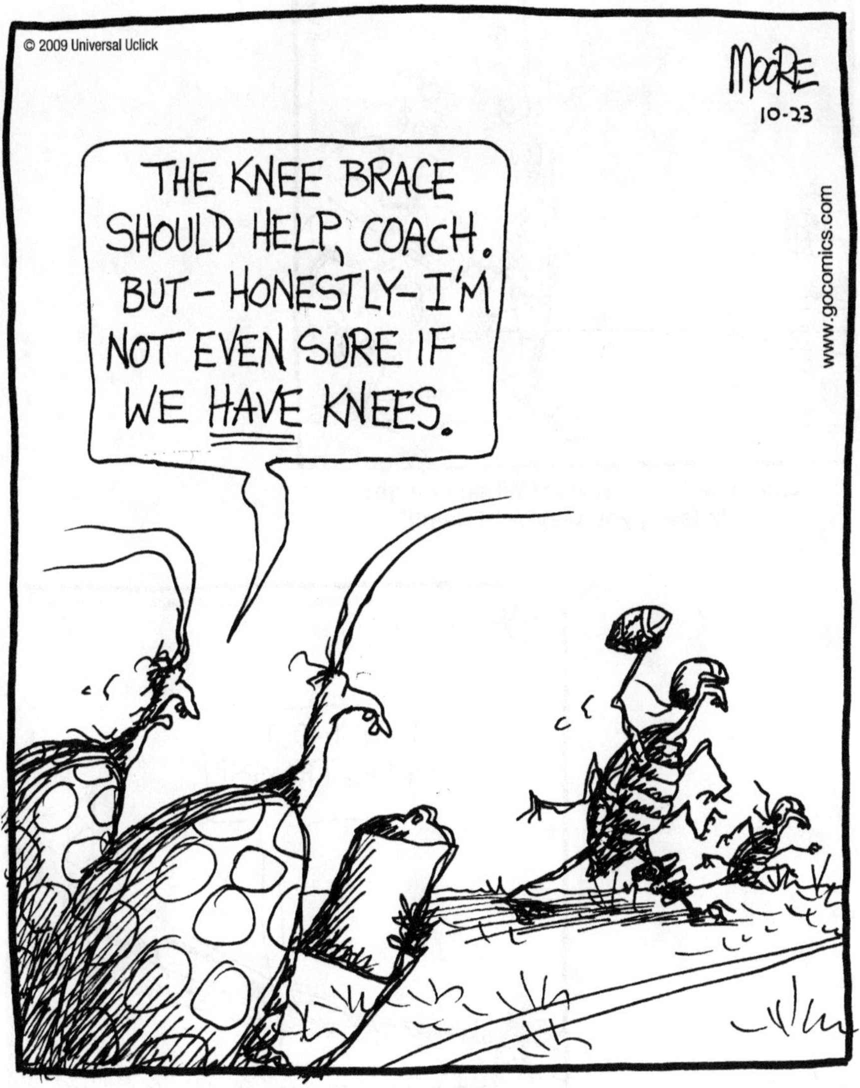
© 2009 Universal Uclick
MOORE
10-23
www.gocomics.com
THE KNEE BRACE SHOULD HELP, COACH. BUT - HONESTLY - I'M NOT EVEN SURE IF WE HAVE KNEES.

MOORE
4/22
In the Bleachers © 2011 Steve Moore. Dist. by Universal Uclick

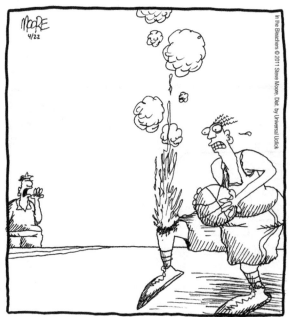

"Quit whining, Johnson! When you get to this level, you play with pain!!"

MOORE
12/17
In the Bleachers © 2010 Steve Moore. Dist. by Universal Uclick
TIME OUT! LEG CRAMPS!!

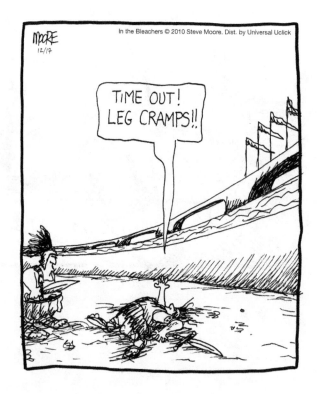

MOORE
10/27
In the Bleachers © 2010 Steve Moore. Dist. by Universal Uclick

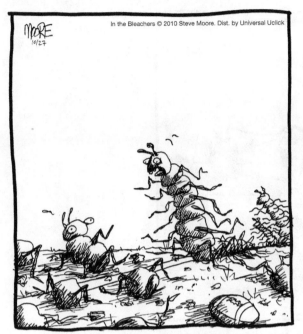

"Don't move, Danny! They're bringing in a neck brace as a precaution."

In the Bleachers © 2011 Steve Moore. Dist. by Universal Uclick
MOORE
4/23

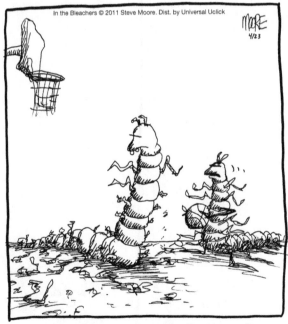

"The legs are always the first to go."

MOORE
12/15
In the Bleachers © 2010 Steve Moore. Dist. by Universal Uclick
GRIT
TRUE GRIT

"Not that ... Fill him up with the *good* stuff!"

MOORE
3/12
In the Bleachers © 2011 Steve Moore. Dist. by Universal Uclick
STUPIDLY PASSED UP NFL DRAFT TO PLAY SENIOR YEAR

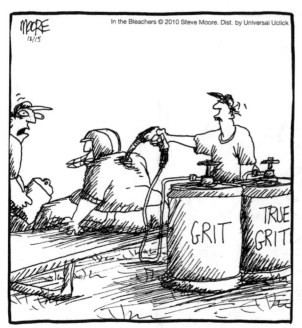

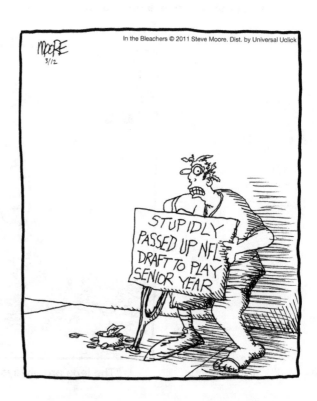

© 2010 Universal Uclick www.gocomics.com
MOORE
10/8

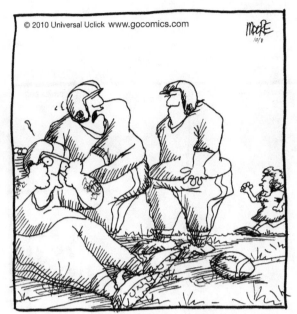

"It's serious! He hurt his feelings and ... oh, thank God. Here comes his mom."

In the Bleachers © 2010 Steve Moore. Dist. by Universal Uclick
MOORE
10/11
PERSONAL FOUL... PECKING AT AN OPEN WOUND... FIFTEEN YARDS!

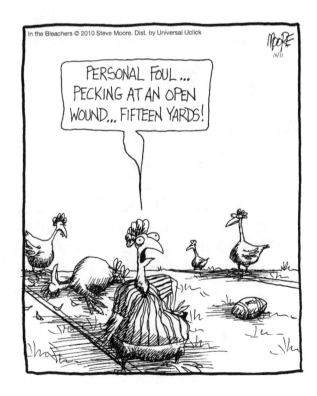

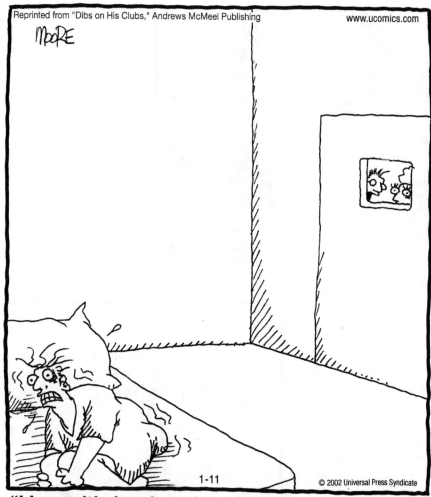

Reprinted from "Dibs on His Clubs," Andrews McMeel Publishing
www.ucomics.com
MOORE
1-11
© 2002 Universal Press Syndicate

"I know it's hard, ma'am, but the worst is over. The vomiting and severe shakes are nearly gone, and soon your husband's body will no longer crave golf."

© 2010 Universal Uclick www.gocomics.com
WHERE AM I? HOW DID I GET HERE? WHEN CAN I GO HOME?
YOU'VE GOT A DISLOCATED SHOULDER.
MOORE 10/7

In the Bleachers © 2014 Steve Moore. Dist. by Universal Uclick
www.gocomics.com/inthebleachers
MOORE 11/14
THE END OF YOUR CAREER IS NEAR!

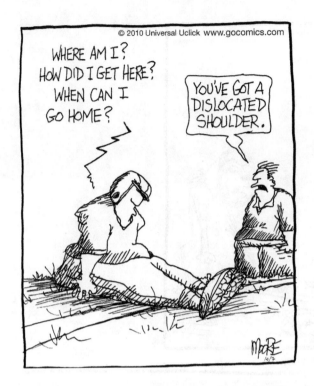

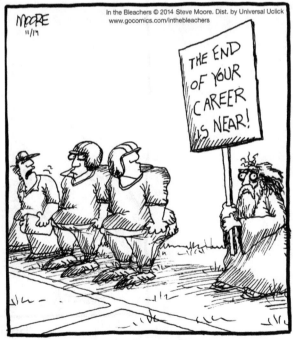

"Get him off the field!!"

MOORE 11/1
In the Bleachers © 2014 Steve Moore. Dist. by Universal Uclick
www.gocomics.com/inthebleachers

"Jock rash."

In the Bleachers © 2014 Steve Moore. Dist. by Universal Uclick
www.gocomics.com/inthebleachers
MOORE 8/12

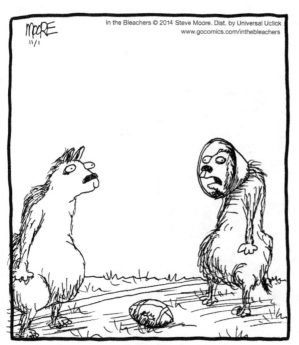

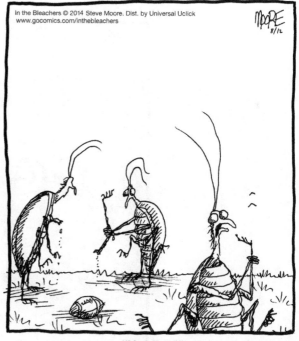

"Holding!"

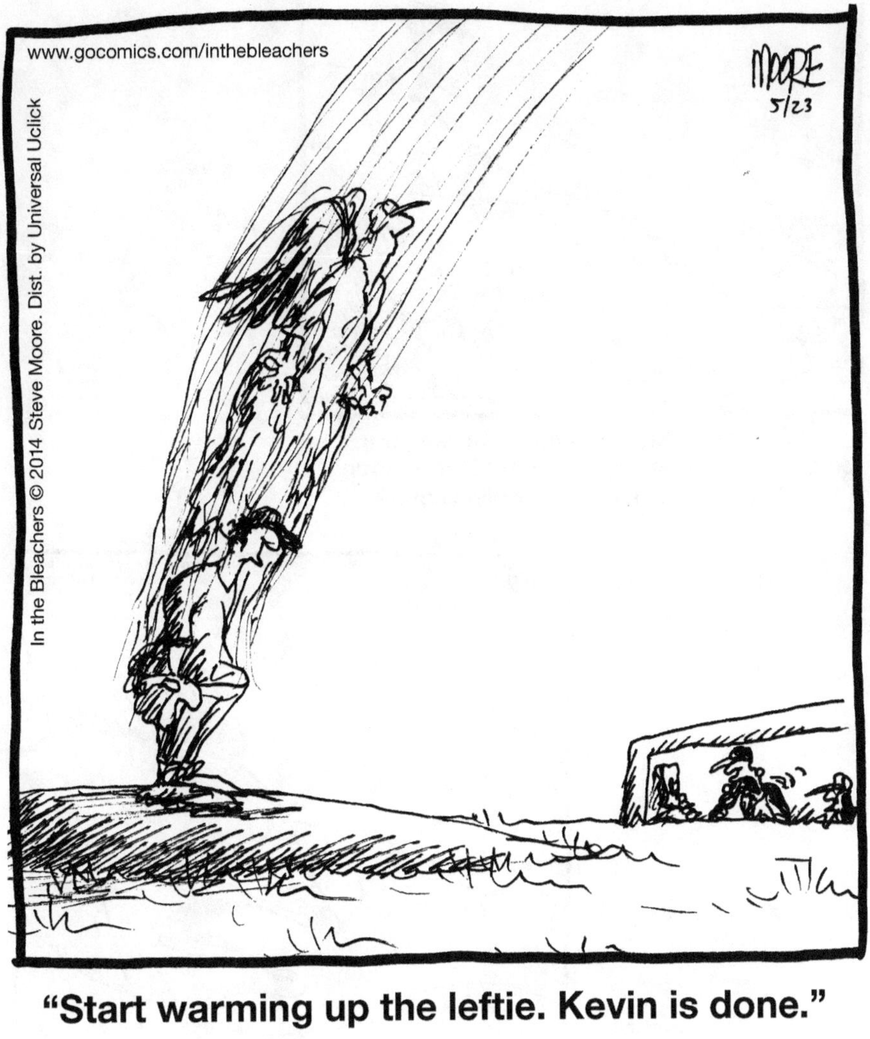
www.gocomics.com/inthebleachers
MOORE
5/23

"Start warming up the leftie. Kevin is done."

MOORE
11/26
In the Bleachers © 2014 Steve Moore. Dist. by Universal Uclick
www.gocomics.com/inthebleachers

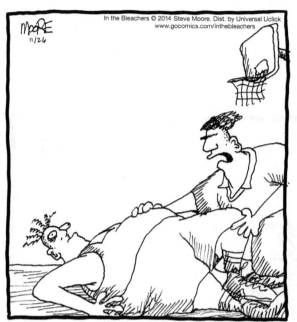

"You tore a knee ligament, broke your collarbone and snapped an Achilles tendon ... No worries. I've got Gorilla Glue!!"

MOORE
4/30
In the Bleachers © 2014 Steve Moore. Dist. by Universal Uclick
www.gocomics.com/inthebleachers

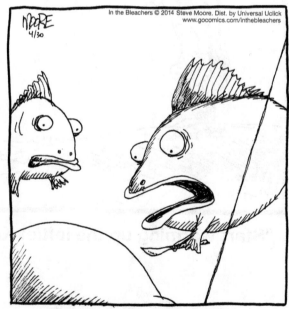

"There it is ... Whoa! He swallowed the hook, line and — talk about gullible! He also swallowed the sinker!!"

In the Bleachers © 2014 Steve Moore. Dist. by Universal Uclick
www.gocomics.com/inthebleachers
MOORE
11/10

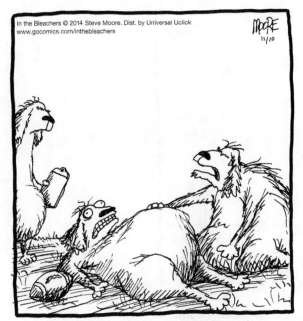

"It's a tummy ache. Once he scarfs some grass and regurgitates, he'll be right back on the field."

In the Bleachers © 2016 Steve Moore. Dist. by Universal Uclick 7/1
www.gocomics.com/inthebleachers
MOORE

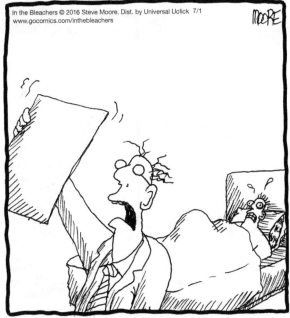

"It's not good. The only athletic bone in your entire body has been shattered into a thousand pieces."

In the Bleachers © 2016 Steve Moore. Dist. by Universal Uclick 8/19
www.gocomics.com/inthebleachers
MOORE

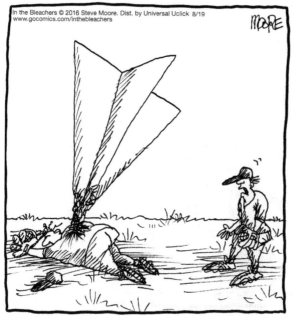

"Get up, Dewey. It's just a paper airplane tossed from the upper deck ... Dewey?"

MOORE
In the Bleachers © 2016 Steve Moore. Dist. by Universal Uclick 7/4
www.gocomics.com/inthebleachers

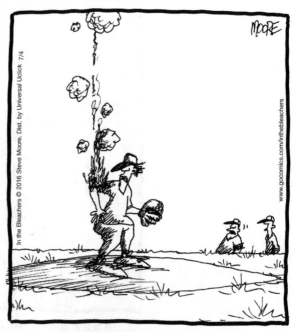

"Maybe 325 pitches in a single game were too many."

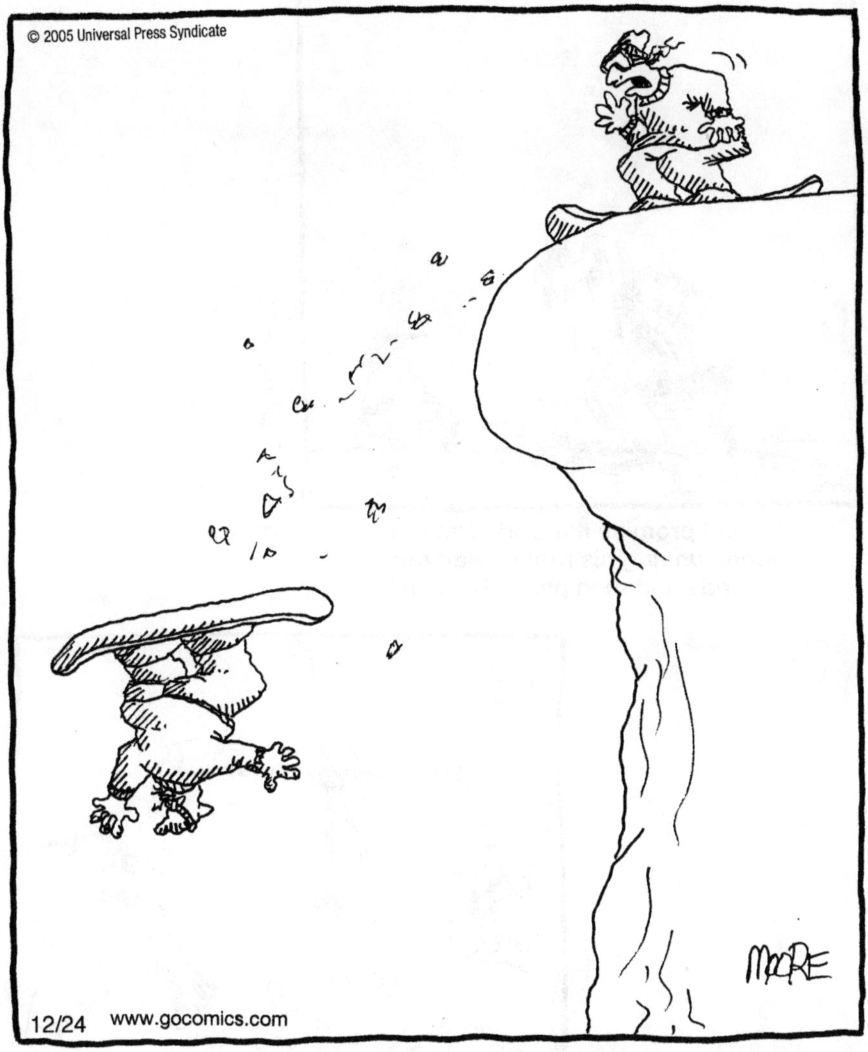

© 2005 Universal Press Syndicate
12/24 www.gocomics.com
MOORE

“Good! And now — by simply shifting your weight — begin to carve a wide, slow turn across the slope.”

In the Bleachers © 2016 Steve Moore. Dist. by Universal Uclick 9/3
www.gocomics.com/inthebleachers
MOORE

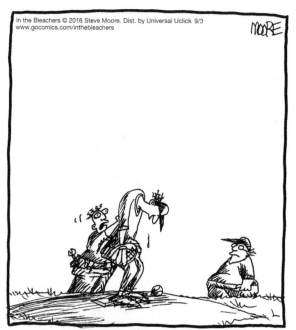

"I can't promise it'll work. But I'm gonna unplug his router, wait ten seconds and then plug it back in."

© 2009 Universal Press Syndicate
MOORE
6-29
www.gocomics.com

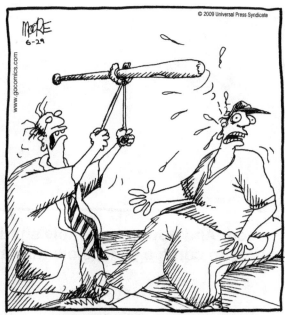

"Got it! Next time, Mr. Blake, use a cotton swab to get at the earwax."

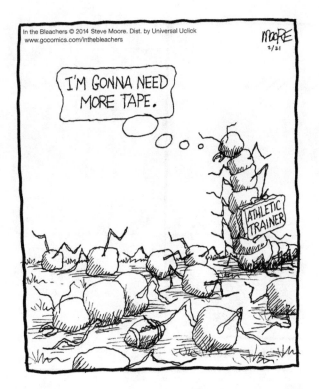

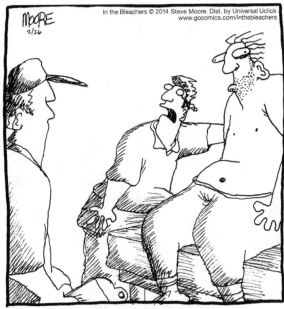

"I checked vital signs, screened for
concussion and took X-rays ... But it
turns out he's just a crybaby."

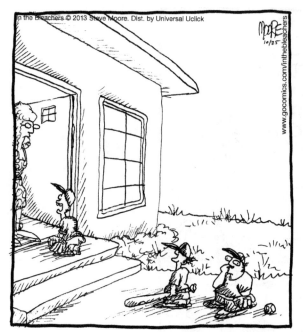

"Hi! Can Alex come out and take steroids?"

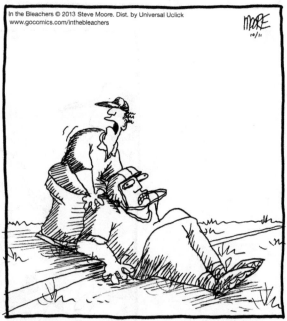

"Too much gluten! ... Get a stretcher!!"

In the Bleachers © 2014 Steve Moore. Dist. by Universal Uclick
www.gocomics.com/inthebleachers
MOORE
3/19

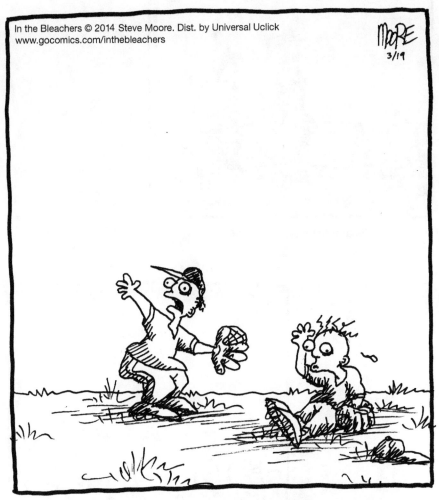

"Time out! Billy just got hit with puberty!!"

www.gocomics.com/inthebleachers
MOORE
9/26
In the Bleachers © 2013 Steve Moore. Dist. by Universal Uclick

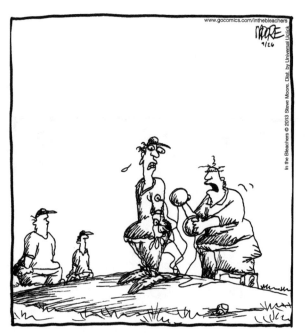

"His arm flat-lined ... CLEAR!!"

In the Bleachers © 2013 Steve Moore. Dist. by Universal Uclick
www.gocomics.com/inthebleachers
MOORE
10/4

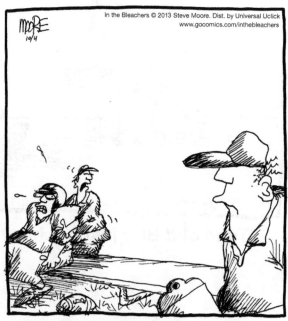

"There's no concussion, but the blow reignited a deep-rooted hatred of his ex-wife!!"

In the Bleachers © 2013 Steve Moore. Dist. by Universal Uclick
www.gocomics.com/inthebleachers
MOORE
11/11

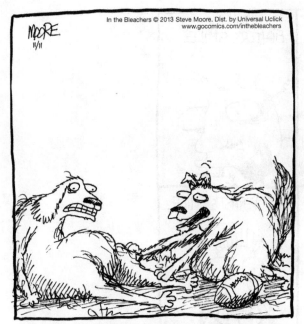

"Oh, this is bad! We're gonna need to put you to sleep! ... Kidding! It's just a sprain."

In the Bleachers © 2013 Steve Moore. Dist. by Universal Uclick
www.gocomics.com/inthebleachers
MOORE
9/9

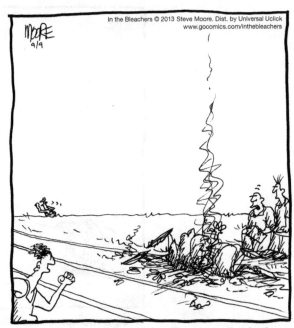

"We should put up a sign: Counter-clockwise. Always counter-clockwise."

HOCKEY PLAYER'S SMILE
ULTIMATE FIGHTER'S SMILE
RUGBY PLAYER'S SMILE
THEIR DENTIST'S SMILE
In the Bleachers © 2013 Steve Moore. Dist. by Universal Uclick
www.gocomics.com/inthebleachers
MOORE 12/4

In the Bleachers © 2013 Steve Moore. Dist. by Universal Uclick
www.gocomics.com/inthebleachers
MOORE 11/2

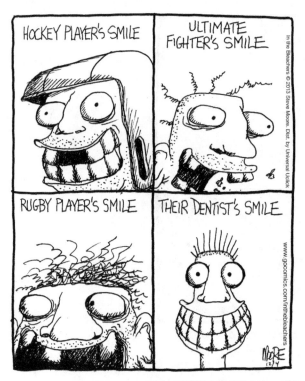

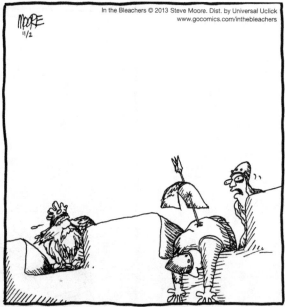

"It's a message from the battlefield, majesty. Our men claim that their helmets offer only minimal protection against concussions!"

In the Bleachers © 2013 Steve Moore. Dist. by Universal Uclick
www.gocomics.com/inthebleachers
MOORE 11/25
• WHAT IS THE NATURE OF THE UNIVERSE?
• HOW DID IT COME TO EXIST?
• WHAT IS ITS PURPOSE?

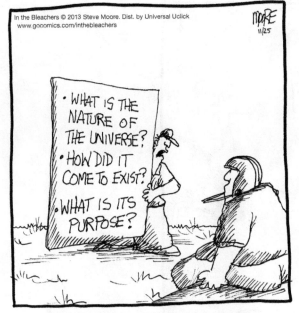

"You took a hard blow to the head. I'll tell coach you're OK to go back in the game if you can answer these three simple questions correctly."

MOORE 11/20
In the Bleachers © 2013 Steve Moore. Dist. by Universal Uclick
www.gocomics.com/inthebleachers
I KNOW THE PROCEDURE IS RUNNING LONG! BUT STOP REFERRING TO IT AS 'SUDDEN-DEATH OVERTIME'...!!

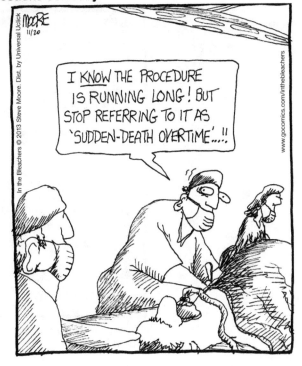

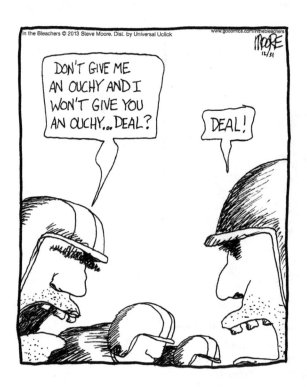

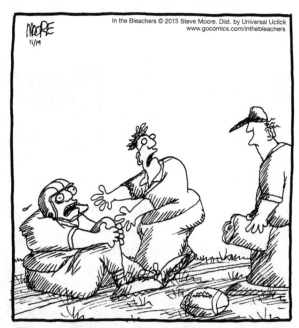

"We won't know until the MRI, but I'm certain that it's either an 'ouchie' or a 'boo-boo' ..."

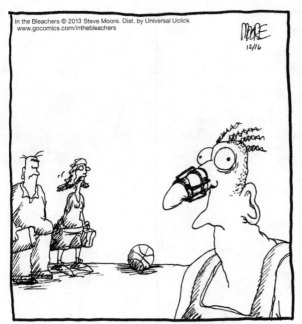

"It's just a bad sprain, so he can
play if he wears the nose brace."

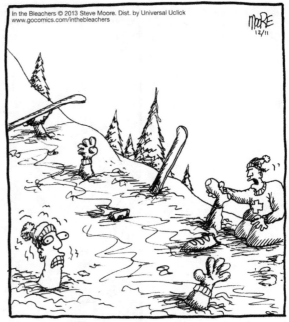

"Can you wiggle your toes?"

© 1996 Universal Press Syndicate
MOORE
9-27
THIS BRACE WILL HELP YOUR BRAIN WITH BASIC, DAY-TO-DAY DECISIONS... BUT YOUR PLAYING DAYS ARE OVER, PAL.

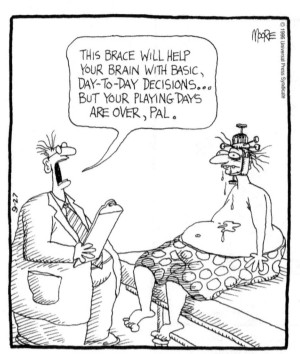

Another career-ending chess injury.

In the Bleachers © 2013 Steve Moore. Dist. by Universal Uclick
www.gocomics.com/inthebleachers
MOORE
8/9
OL' LUKE IS EXCITED! YOUR BOY MUST HAVE GOT HIMSELF A REEEEAL DOOZIE!!

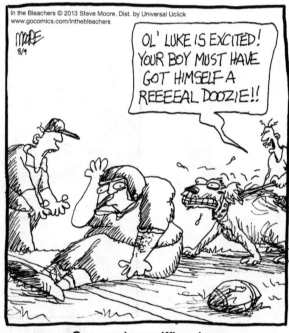

Concussion-sniffing dogs.

In the Bleachers © 2013 Steve Moore. Dist. by Universal Uclick
www.gocomics.com/inthebleachers
MOORE 9/5
OH, THAT'S A BAD ONE!
I'M GONNA BE SICK!
TIME OUT!! HANSEN'S GOT A HANGNAIL!!

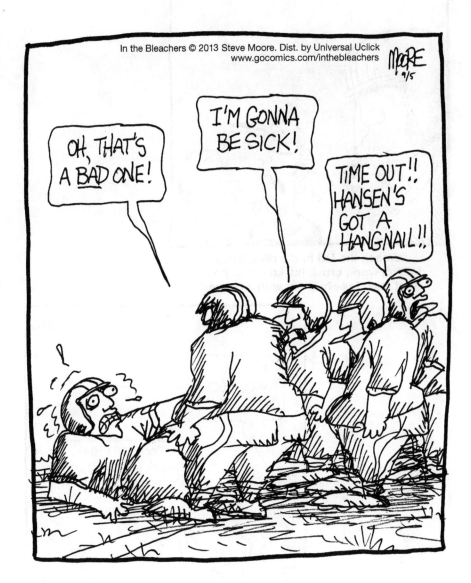

In the Bleachers © 2013 Steve Moore. Dist. by Universal Uclick
www.gocomics.com/inthebleachers
MOORE
9/10

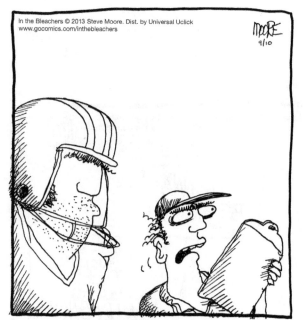

"Smash the QB in the ribs. If that doesn't work, crush his knees ... And if that fails, take him out with a drone."

© 2005 Universal Press Syndicate
MOORE
IT'S HIS ANKLE - GET SOME ICE!!
TOO LATE! RUN! SHE'S GONNA BLOW!!
4-4
www.ucomics.com

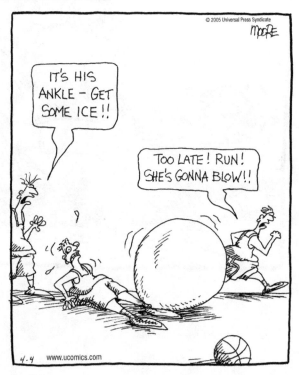

12/9 MOORE
© 1995 Universal Press Syndicate

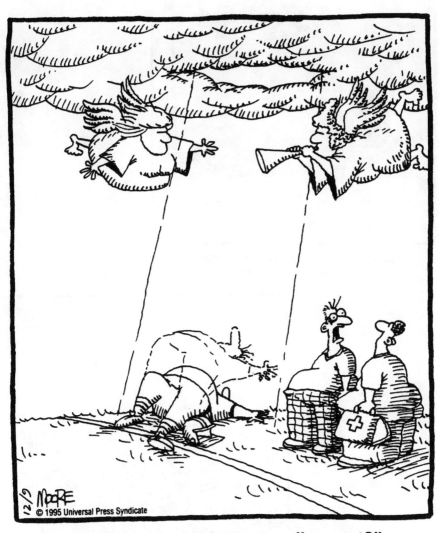

"Are you sure it's just a torn ligament?"

© 2000 Universal Press Syndicate
www.uexpress.com
MOORE
2-25

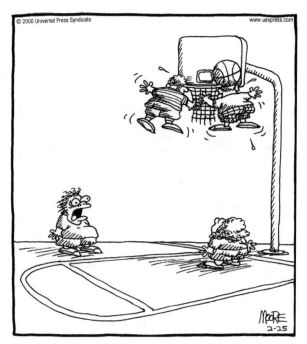

"Well, now Tommy, Kyle *and* the ball are stuck. You'd better go get your dad."

MOORE
2-8
© 2000 Universal Press Syndicate
www.uexpress.com

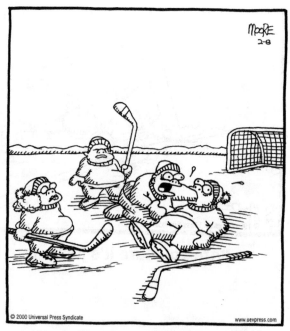

"I give up. It's just out of reach. Someone run and fetch another puck."

© 2001 Universal Press Syndicate
www.ucomics.com
I WIN!!
LIFE
FINISH LINE
MOORE
5-16

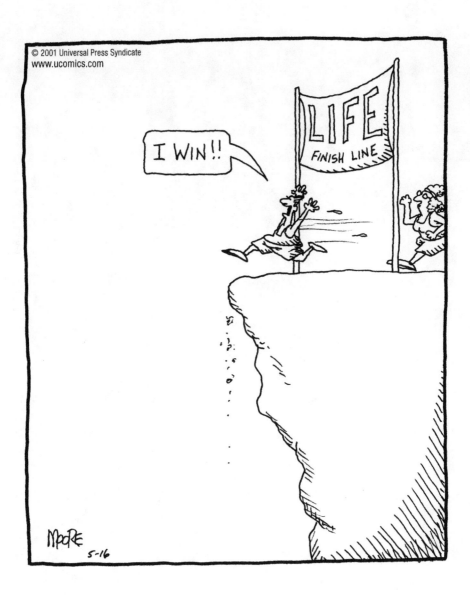

About the Cartoonist

STEVE MOORE is a syndicated cartoonist, children's book author and creator and writer of animated feature films.

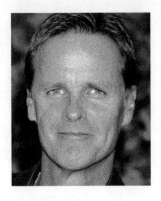

In 1985, Moore created *In the Bleachers*, a comic distributed worldwide by Andrews McMeel Syndication. In 2016, Moore reluctantly handed off his *Bleachers* comic due to Essential Tremor, a neurological disability that causes shaking in the hands. (Cartoons in this book were curated from Moore's archive of more than 11,000 drawings that he created from 1985 to 2016.)

Moore also is author and illustrator of *King of the Bench*, a series of middle-grade novels published by HarperCollins.

In film, he teamed up with Oscar-winning *Rango* producer John Carls to create, write the original story and serve as Exec. Producer for *Open Season*, Sony Pictures Animation's first feature film. Moore also was creator, writer and producer of the animated movie *Alpha & Omega* for Lionsgate Films.

He is a former Exec. News Editor for the *Los Angeles Times*. Moore graduated from Oregon State University and received a Masters degree in Journalism & Communications from the University of Oregon.

Moore grew up in La Canada Flintridge, California. He has three grown children - Jakob, Lauren and Chris - and lives in Idaho with his wife, Melaine, a parrot named Ulu and a hilarious snake named Tiny Fey.

In college, Moore snapped ACLs in both his knees. The joints have since been replaced with some kind of artificial gizmos.

In the Bleachers © 2014 Steve Moore. Dist. by Universal Uclick
www.gocomics.com/inthebleachers
MOORE
2/10
ATHLETIC TRAINER

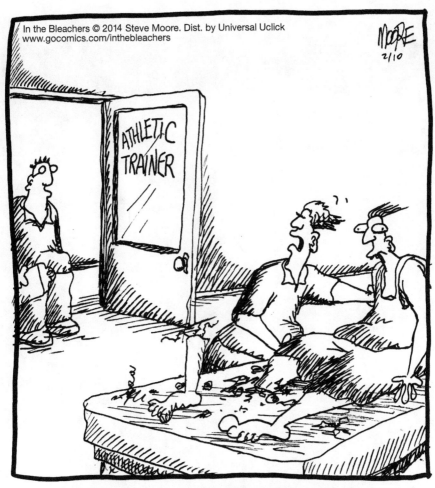

"Knees are complicated, coach. I took a look 'under the hood' and he needs a couple of replacement gizmos before he can go back in the game."

Other Creations by

MOORE

My name is Steve,
and I'm the king of the bench!
You might be wondering why I'd write a book and tell total strangers all about being a benchwarmer and the humiliating phobia that almost ruined my first year on the baseball team.
Duh. It's pretty much a rule that you spill your guts when you write a book about yourself.
So go ahead, open it. Just don't tell anyone what really happened with that snake.
US $13.99 / $17.50 CAN
HARPER
MOORE
KING of the BENCH
NO FEAR!
VOL. 1
HARPER
KING of the BENCH
NO FEAR!
STEVE MOORE

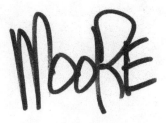

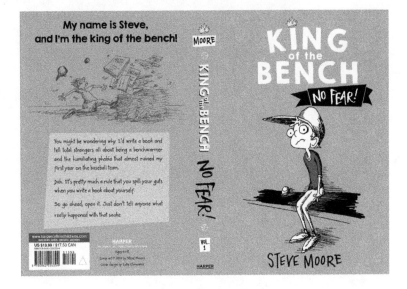

KING OF THE BENCH: The critically acclaimed HarperCollins series of middle-grade novels with cartoons, starring an extraordinarily average 12 year-old who plays the same position in every sport … bench-warmer.

For ages 7 to 12
Available at Amazon Books, Barnes & Noble,
HarperCollins Publishing

And Coming Soon ...

IT ONLY LAUGHS WHEN I HURT

Another

IN THE BLEACHERS

Collection of Painfully Funny Sports Injury Cartoons

(Vol. 2)